"A masterful blending of play therapy theories and techniques in make-believe play sessions. Thought-provoking and insightful!"
Charles Schaefer, Ph.D., Registered Play Therapy Supervisor,
Co-Founder & Director Emeritus,
The Association for Play Therapy, USA

"*Integrative Play Therapy with Individuals, Families and Groups* provides a comprehensive blueprint to guide both beginners and seasoned practitioners. Ariel methodically links concepts from systems, linguistic and play theory to create an innovative, integrated approach to diagnosis and treatment, the Diamond Model. The application of the model is illustrated though compelling and in-depth case examples in varying treatment formats. The practice of integrative play therapy is further exhibited by thought-provoking dialogues about the cases with an interdisciplinary team. The complexity of issues confronting practitioners today is daunting. Ariel's book offers a theoretically grounded, methodical and thorough guide to construct effective and playful interventions."
Professor Anne Stewart, Department of Graduate Psychology,
James Madison University, Harrisonburg, Virginia,
Member of the Association for Play Therapy Board of Directors,
Past President of the Virginia Association for Play Therapy, USA

"Once again, Dr. Ariel has challenged and articulated insights into our play therapy field. Words like preparatory moves, integration of family and individual therapy, interdisciplinary approaches and collaborative supervision come alive in this, his most recent book. Such a pleasure in our times to hear from a clinician with wisdom, not just knowledge, but wisdom with respect to the entire child and his/her family."
Allan Gonsher, L.C.S.W., Registered Play Therapy Supervisor,
Founder and Chief Executive Officer, Kids Inc., USA

Integrative Play Therapy with Individuals, Families and Groups

Integrative Play Therapy with Individuals, Families and Groups is a complete theory-to-practice introduction to a comprehensive integrative model of play therapy, developed by Shlomo Ariel. It synthesizes numerous concepts, methods and techniques found in the various branches of play theory and research under a unified conceptual and linguistic roof of information-processing, cybernetics and semiotics. The author's tenet is that any case, whatever the presenting difficulties, can be treated by such an integrative, multi-systemic approach.

This book abounds with vivid observations and case descriptions, followed by discussions in a fictional interdisciplinary seminar. Every chapter is followed by a brief summary, homework assignments and a classified list of relevant publications.

Integrative Play Therapy with Individuals, Families and Groups will generate immense interest throughout the play therapy community. It can serve as a textbook for budding play therapists and as a reference book for more experienced practitioners.

Shlomo Ariel is an Israeli senior clinical psychologist and family therapist, widely published in his areas of expertise – psychotherapy integration, play research, play therapy and culturally competent psychotherapy. He is an international trainer of therapists in these areas.

Integrative Play Therapy with Individuals, Families and Groups

Shlomo Ariel

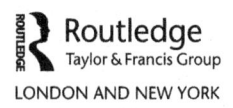

Routledge
Taylor & Francis Group
LONDON AND NEW YORK

Disclaimer: The cases included in this book are inspired by real cases, but the crucial details have been altered to the point that they are not recognizable and any remaining likeness to the original cases is entirely coincidental.

First published 2019
by Routledge
2 Park Square, Milton Park, Abingdon, Oxon OX14 4RN

and by Routledge
52 Vanderbilt Avenue, New York, NY 10017

Routledge is an imprint of the Taylor & Francis Group, an informa business

© 2019 Shlomo Ariel

The right of Shlomo Ariel to be identified as author of this work has been asserted by him in accordance with sections 77 and 78 of the Copyright, Designs and Patents Act 1988.

All rights reserved. No part of this book may be reprinted or reproduced or utilised in any form or by any electronic, mechanical, or other means, now known or hereafter invented, including photocopying and recording, or in any information storage or retrieval system, without permission in writing from the publishers.

Trademark notice: Product or corporate names may be trademarks or registered trademarks, and are used only for identification and explanation without intent to infringe.

British Library Cataloguing-in-Publication Data
A catalogue record for this book is available from the British Library

Library of Congress Cataloging-in-Publication Data
Names: Ariel, Shlomo, author.
Title: Integrative play therapy with individuals, families and groups/Shlomo Ariel.
Description: Milton Park, Abingdon, Oxon; New York, NY: Routledge, 2019. | Includes bibliographical references and index.
Identifiers: LCCN 2019001327 (print) | LCCN 2019009024 (ebook) | ISBN 9780429198151 (Master e-Book) | ISBN 9780367187675 (hardback: alk. paper) | ISBN 9780367187682 (pbk.: alk. paper) | ISBN 9780429198151 (ebk)
Subjects: LCSH: Play therapy. | Family psychotherapy. | Group psychotherapy.
Classification: LCC RJ505.P6 (ebook) | LCC RJ505.P6 A74 2019 (print) | DDC 618.92/891653--dc23
LC record available at https://lccn.loc.gov/2019001327

ISBN: 978-0-367-18767-5 (hbk)
ISBN: 978-0-367-18768-2 (pbk)
ISBN: 978-0-429-19815-1 (ebk)

Typeset in Times New Roman
by Deanta Global Publishing Services, Chennai, India

Printed in the United Kingdom
by Henry Ling Limited

Contents

Preface	ix
Acknowledgments	xi
Introduction	1

PART 1
Theoretical and methodological foundations — 3

1	My favorite play therapy mix	5
2	Appraising the current state of the art	12
3	The Diamond Model	19

PART 2
X-raying make-believe play — 35

4	Play observation techniques	37
5	Microscopic analysis of observed play	42
6	Macroscopic analysis on the semantic level	47
7	Macroscopic analysis on the pragmatic level	56

PART 3
The manifold magic of make-believe play — 65

8	A formal definition of make-believe play	67
9	Linguistic peculiarities of make-believe play	81

10	Make-believe play as a vehicle of learning and development	88
11	Make-believe play as a pacifier	96
12	The therapeutic powers of play, revisited	108

PART 4
Planning a multi-systemic play therapy — 117

13	Multi-systemic diagnostic evaluation	119
14	Planning a therapeutic strategy	140

PART 5
How to do it? — 145

15	Conducting a play-therapeutic session	147
16	Lucy: the girl who created her own father	163
17	Nadav: a sweet oppositional-defiant boy	177
18	Play therapy: a reality show	207
19	Finale	213

List of cases, sessions and observations — 217
Index — 219

Preface

Since I became a parent, I have never stopped being fascinated by children. They have the naïve curiosity of the greatest inventors and scientists, who take nothing for granted. They can ask, like Newton, why an apple falls from the tree down and not sideways or up. They invent creative ideas, intriguing even if bizarre, such as that body heat can bake bread from flour and water inside the stomach. They make statements like, "Horses cannot have a flat tire". In their imaginative play, they effortlessly create images such as a baby dragon shedding tears of fire over a pet cockroach, grabbed by another baby dragon in the dragons' nursery school. They can play Poohsticks for hours.

That insatiable fascination and curiosity had motivated me to spend a prominent part of my professional life exploring the inner world and behavior of children, especially as these are expressed in their individual and social make-believe play. I soon came to realize that my former background in theoretical and anthropological linguistics, child language development, semiotics and cognitive science had equipped me with invaluable tools for this endeavor.

Later in my career I was trained as a clinical psychologist and family therapist. I began to apply the results of my explorations in my practice with individual children, children's peer groups and families. I was concerned about the fact that it was difficult if not impossible to involve little children significantly in family therapy. Since I had not found a solution to this difficulty in the professional literature, I set about developing a model that systematically integrates family therapy with play therapy. This model, first published in 1992 in my book, *Strategic Family Play Therapy*, has served as a source in various international training programs.

When I started my career as a play therapist, that discipline was not as highly developed and multifaceted as it is today. Even though play has always been the primary tool for child therapy, most child therapists were mainly applying concepts and techniques developed by old-school psychoanalysts. Axline's child-centered, non-directive play therapy began to have an impact as well. Since then, the field of play therapy has grown and expanded immeasurably. Scores of play therapy theoretical models and methodologies have been sprouting and growing rapidly. Play-therapeutic techniques have been specially designed to treat specific syndromes. Other models and techniques of family play therapy have been proposed, in addition to methods of group play therapy. Serious attempts have been made to base play therapy on concepts and findings of play research, developmental psychology, neuropsychology and other disciplines. Ways have been proposed to blend and integrate various models and methods of play therapy.

This dizzying wealth of approaches is impressive, but can also be confusing, especially for early stage therapists. At least some major parts of it can be assembled under a single theoretical and methodological roof, cleaned up so to speak, explicated, simplified, formalized and systematized. The results of my efforts to achieve such an integration are presented in this book.

Acknowledgments

Of the many individuals who have contributed to this work, directly or indirectly, I would like to express my special thanks to the following persons:

In 1979, I was invited by Professor Jerome L. Singer to participate in his play research in the Psychology Department at Yale University. I am deeply indebted to Professor Singer not just for the opportunity to have direct access to his pioneering, highly inspiring work on play, but also for his personal support and encouragement.

I must also mention the late Professor Brian Sutton-Smith, with whom I had long-term exchanges, and who wrote an insightful foreword to my book, *Children's Imaginative Play: A Visit to Wonderland*.

I would like to express my gratitude to Professor Charles Schaefer, "the father of play therapy", who has supported my work on play therapy in various ways, including endorsing this book.

I'm grateful to Professor Anne Stewart, a colleague and a friend, for having read the manuscript and submitted her endorsement.

My colleague and friend Dr. Odeda Peled has been my play therapy mate for many years. I have learned a lot from her creative work with children who suffer from developmental and communication difficulties.

I am deeply indebted to Allan Gonsher, founder and director of Kids Inc and a highly esteemed practitioner and teacher of play therapy, for his unbending support and encouragement.

I am thankful to my wife Ruti and my daughter Nana for their merciless, insightful and highly instructive critiques of my work.

My children, grandchildren and the numerous children I have observed playing and attempted to help by play therapy have been a great source of inspiration for me and taught me everything I know about play.

Introduction

Play is an inexhaustible treasure of magic. A play therapist can be a magician. To master the gold mine of playful magic tricks, a play therapist must acquire a wide range of ways of thinking and skills in a long and complex process of training. This book is intended to serve as a guide in such process of training. It is a complete introduction to integrative, multi-dimensional, individual, family and group play therapy. It leads the reader and learner step-by-step through a clinical understanding of a case, planning the therapy and carrying it out by means of play as a primary therapeutic tool. All these stages are informed by the Diamond Model, developed by the author and published in his book, *Multi-Dimensional Therapy with Families Children and Adults: The Diamond Model* (published by Routledge in 2018). The Diamond Model constitutes an attempt to lay a solid theoretical and methodological foundation for psychotherapy in general, but this book emphasizes its application in understanding play and its therapeutic powers.

The first part of the book lays the theoretical and methodological foundations of the author's approach to integrative play therapy. A play therapist is advised to stand onstage rather than just sit in the hall as an audience, to be an active partner in the spontaneous play of the client(s) rather than an external reflector, interpreter or director. It is argued that the compartmentalization of play therapy into distinct approaches such as psychodynamic, cognitive-behavioral, systemic, etc. is arbitrary. All these approaches can be incorporated in a grand theory of play and multi-dimensional play therapy. It is also contended that different types of difficulties such as PTSD, conduct disorders, anxiety disorders, etc. should not be treated by different play therapy methods, but by the same multi-dimensional, integrative method. This is followed by some critical comments on the current relevant literature. It should be emphasized though that no complete literature review is attempted. Ways are proposed to base the current play therapy approaches on a firm theoretical and methodological basis. The basics of the Diamond Model are presented briefly.

The second part of the book is devoted to methods and techniques of recording, analyzing and interpreting observed make-believe play as a semiotic, information-processing and cybernetic system. Spontaneous individual, family and group play behaviors, before and during play therapy sessions, are recorded and analyzed as sources of multi-dimensional diagnostic information. The analysis of the play data, in addition to data collected from other sources, provides a comprehensive, multi-dimensional picture of the level of functioning of each client. This picture also includes a multi-dimensional developmental profile of each client. This mosaic serves as the knowledge base for planning and carrying out the therapy.

The third part is devoted to methods and techniques of planning the therapy. Principles for designing an overall therapeutic strategy and planning a session are proposed.

In the fourth part, the healing properties of play are examined. The magical therapeutic powers of play are logically derived from the very definition of the concept of make-believe play, from its peculiar linguistic and semiotic characteristics and from its role as a mechanism for achieving emotional and interpersonal balance. Play is also a vehicle of learning and development. A brief critical review of recent work on the therapeutic powers of play is presented.

The fifth and final part proposes methods and techniques of joining the clients' play and conducting individual, family and group play therapy sessions, monitoring and evaluating the therapeutic process and termination. Some cases are presented and analyzed in detail.

The book is filled with numerous vivid observations, case examples and case vignettes. It includes also some dialogues with fictitious trainees, who share their insights, their queries and their difficulties and do not hesitate to argue with the trainer. Each chapter is followed by a brief summary, homework assignments and a classified list of some relevant publications.

This book can serve as a training textbook for budding mental health professionals who work with children, their families and their peers, and as a reference book for experienced clinicians.

Part I

Theoretical and methodological foundations

Chapter 1

My favorite play therapy mix

The kind of play therapy I espouse has the following attributes:

(a) It is not informed by a single theory (psychoanalytic, cognitive-behavioral, systemic, etc.) but by a synthesis of many theories. Every case is multi-faceted, having dark corners and blind alleys into which different theories turn their selective spotlights. All these theories can be synthesized in such a way that the spotlights would be directed at all the relevant corners and alleys.
(b) It follows from the above assertion, that the play therapy (or, for that matter, any therapy) with each case should not be restricted to one setting. Individual, family and group play therapy can be conducted with the same case, simultaneously or in sequence.
(c) It also follows from the above assertions that different kinds of difficulties and syndromes should not necessarily be treated by play-therapeutic or other methods specially designed to tackle a specific kind of presenting problem. Every set of symptoms, e.g. post-traumatic stress disorder, phobias, depression, conduct disorders, etc., is multi-determined. It is the product of a complex interaction between genetic and developmental agents, personality traits, conscious and unconscious conflictual cognitive and emotional processes, life events and circumstances, family and social dynamics, culture, ecology, etc. Therefore, any suitable play-therapeutic methods and techniques can be used with any kind of presenting difficulties. The choice of play-therapeutic vehicles is governed by a deep understanding of the case, not just by focusing on the external symptoms. Such understanding is achieved by a multi-systemic diagnostic assessment.

One might argue against this approach that, considering studies that have proven the efficacy of target-oriented, evidence-based play-therapeutic (and other) treatment methods, the best choice would be applying just such proven methods in working with each case. For example, play-therapeutic methods using habituation, catharsis and abreaction have been found to be effective in treating post-traumatic stress disorder. Cognitive-behavioral play therapy has been shown to be effective in treating obsessive-compulsive disorder.

6 Theoretical and methodological foundations

Theraplay has been found to be useful in treating reactive attachment disorder. My view is: All these studies are based just on statistical generalizations. They cannot take into account the totality of the factors that affect the difficulties in each specific case. Indeed, it is useful to use proven techniques, but only as part of a treatment plan tailored specifically for each case.

(d) A play therapist is not just a reflecting or interpreting observer of the clients' play. She is an active participant in the individual, group or family's spontaneous play. As an active participant, she is an equal partner and a co-creator of the clients' play. The play therapist can still reflect on or interpret the clients' play, but as an insider with a make-believe role.

Here are some of the reasons why I prefer such active involvement: In most cases, play is a private, intimate, sometimes secretive activity. Group play is also a private activity, shared only by the group members. In many cases players do not want a stranger, even if the stranger is a play therapist, to watch their play and comment on it. They feel this to be as intrusion into their private domain during their intimate moments. I have often witnessed children in play therapy hiding underneath a table or behind big pillows to prevent the therapist from prying into their play, meddling with it and knowing what it is about. Many children are happy to share their play with the therapist only if he has been admitted to their play as a partner, on their own terms. Furthermore, the therapist's tracking, reflections and interpretations are usually wasted on the players, because they are too absorbed in their own play to listen and even more so to process what they have heard. True, there are quite a few cases in which children play for the therapist as audience, like actors on stage. I do not claim that such a show is never of any therapeutic value, but sometimes it is no more than showing off, with the truly important contents left unexpressed.

Another advantage of the therapist's active participation in the clients' play is the wealth of therapeutic means that can be applied, and the great flexibility made possible. Play in general and make-believe play in particular are singularly rich and flexible media of expression and communication. Play speaks through words, actions, objects and materials. Roles and modes of behavior can be flexibly changed at will. An unlimited number of events and situations can be made up freely. A creative therapist who actively participates in the clients' play can invent a great variety of therapeutic moves. She may choose positions such as "a script writer", "a producer", "a director", "an actor", "a stage manager", "a stage designer", "a musician" and so on. As an actor, the therapist can play various roles such as "the dangerous monster" or "the submissive sheep". She can roll on the carpet, dance, sing, shout, cry, laugh, do pantomime, wear various hats and masks, change costumes and fancy dresses, what not. And above all, playing is great fun, much more so than sitting on the sidelines and making learned comments.

These attributes of my approach can be illustrated by the following case and the ensuing discussion:

Case 1.1 Rusella
Rusella (9) was the laughing-stock of her classmates. They used to call her Miss Piggy and Dummy. She was overweight and had difficulty walking, because of a congenital hip dysplasia. Her habit of deliberately talking in a baby voice definitely did not improve her social situation. The children were mimicking her manners of walking and talking. So were her mother and fourteen-year-old brother, who thought it was funny. But while in school she would respond to the harassment with blows and kicks, at home she would join her mother and brother's laugher when they imitated her, so they saw it as an amusing game that Rusella enjoyed too. Often her mother assigned her the task of taking care of her two-year-old sister. The rest of the time her mother simply ignored her, as if she didn't exist.

Rusella's father left home when she was seven. He was visiting his children at their mother's home irregularly. During visits, the children's parents would behave as if they had never parted. When Rusella's father was around, Rusella would speak with him in what she tried to make sound like a man's voice. She seldom spoke in her normal gender and age-appropriate voice.

Rusella underwent speech therapy that made no difference. She was later referred by her school counselor to the child and adolescent mental health clinic in her home town. The presenting complaint was violence against her female classmates. She was treated individually by Lailah, a clinical psychology intern, under my supervision. Her mother got parental guidance from Daniel, a social work intern, once in two weeks. Her father refused to come to parental guidance.

In the first sessions, Rusella spoke with Lailah in a baby voice, but afterwards began speaking in a normal voice. She told Lailah that even though she was being ridiculed, she felt better about herself when she spoke in a baby voice. Only when she used that voice, she could say whatever came to her mind. She also shared with Lailah that when she was speaking in a baby voice, the children could not understand what she was saying, and that made her feel better. She also said that it was easier for her to talk with her father in a man's voice and was quick to make it clear that she was not at all afraid of her father.

Interdisciplinary seminar

Lailah, Daniel and two other interns – Anna, a creative arts therapist, and Ethan, a school psychologist (the names are fictitious) – participated in an interdisciplinary seminar, under my guidance. The seminar served two purposes: group supervision and being a forum for theoretical and methodological discussions.

In one of the first sessions, Lailah presented Rusella's case. Daniel added information about his parental guidance meetings with Rusella's mother. Here are some verbatim quotes from parts of the discussion:

Lailah: I'll read out to you some parts of my notes:

Session 1.1 Lailah and Rusella

Rusella picks a big gorilla doll and a little rabbit doll and sits on the carpet, not in front of me but at a right angle from me, with the dolls between her legs. She makes the rabbit doll approach the gorilla doll and face it. Then she acts as if the rabbit is saying something, in a loud and angry voice. It was impossible to understand what it was saying, because it spoke gibberish.

I say, "The little rabbit is angry at the gorilla."

Rusella ignores me. She makes the gorilla grab the rabbit and throw it away violently, with a roar.

I say, "O! The gorilla is really angry at the little rabbit!"

Rusella ignores me again. She begins mumbling something, probably gibberish again, in a baby voice, almost whispering. Then she gets up, brings a big teddy- bear, makes the bear slap the gorilla and shout, "Who are you to throw away my rabbit?!"

I didn't respond. I assumed she would ignore my reflections again.

She gets up and gets a woman doll, a girl doll and a baby doll. She approaches me, turns in my direction, hands over to me the woman doll and says, "The mother told the girl to take care of the baby and the girl refused. Then the mother sent the girl away to the forest."

I hold the woman doll and say, "I'm sending you alone to the forest, because you will not take care of your little sister."

I felt awkward. I said it unconvincingly, without effect.

Rusella pulls away from me and takes three girl dolls from the shelf. She holds two dolls in one hand and one doll in the other. The doll she holds in her other hand says to the two dolls, "Do you want to come with me to the forest?"

Each of the two dolls say, "No."

Rusella drops the two dolls to the ground and takes the third doll, the one who had asked the other dolls to come with her to the forest, to the corner of the room, by the desk under which was a waste paper basket. She lays the doll on the carpet and says, "She fell asleep in the forest and the monkeys threw her in the trash."

She throws the doll into the wastepaper basket. She says, "Now she is dead and she is flying in the air."

Shlomo: Lailah, how did you feel when you read this?
Lailah: Now I understood all kinds of things I didn't understand during the session, perhaps because I was too busy thinking about how to react. I understand now that many of the contents she brought to the play reflected the difficulties we discussed earlier. In the graduate play therapy course, we were taught not to interfere actively in the child's play, only to provide a safe environment with minimal limits, track and reflect the contents and feelings expressed in the play. When Rusella gave me a doll and told me to play the mother, I felt uncomfortable. I felt that she wasn't happy with the way I

represented the mother, so she moved away from me and played alone. When I tried to reflect her anger, she ignored me. I had the feeling she did not want me to see her play or interfere.

Shlomo: What you learned in your graduate course was one approach – non-directive, child-centered play therapy. There are many other approaches. I advise therapists to be play partners, co-creators of the clients' play, but this requires training, experience, overcoming shyness and inhibition.

Ethan: I agree. There were so many opportunities to enter the girl's play as a co-player, to delve more deeply into its contents and explore their covert meanings.

Shlomo: Yes, but one should know how to do it. You cannot just barge into the child's play without permission. We'll learn some techniques of how to be admitted to the clients' play.

Daniel: In the play, she spoke in many voices: shouting, roaring, mumbling like a baby and more. She spoke in gibberish. All this corresponds to her use of all kinds of voices in real life, assuming various identities, and taking care not to be understood. If you joined her play and talked to her in voices like hers, you might have found all kinds of things about the meanings and roles of those voices.

Lailah: If…

Ethan: It seems to me that during active participation in the play, one should also pay attention to sharp transitions, transformations, such as that the baby suddenly became a girl. It is parallel to her polyphony, moving between voices.

Anna: I could identify with Rusella's expressions of anger. She allowed herself to take out her pent-up anger by using voice, without resorting to physical violence, because it was "just play".

Ethan: Catharsis, abreaction.

Daniel: In her play she allowed herself not just to express suppressed feelings but also to rebel against the exploitation and abuse that in real life she was co-operating with – to yell at the gorilla, who apparently represented her father, to refuse to take care of her little sister. I'm curious to know who the bear who slapped the gorilla represented.

Lailah: I'm not sure it represented a real person that's actually present in her life. Maybe she created an imaginary figure, symbolizing her wish to have a male parental figure who would protect her against her abusers.

Anna: But even in the imaginary play, she paid the price: To be expelled to the desert, to be thrown, and thrown again and again…

Ethan: In her play she not only was trying to overcome her difficulties. She also reproduced them in the safe environment of the make-believe world: The friends who refused to come with her to the forest, the monkeys who threw her in the trash. In the end she played as if she was dead and floating in the air. This seems to be an expression of death wish or suicidal thoughts.

Lailah: I feel so sorry for her. This is perhaps one of the reasons why I didn't really understand her play during the session. Identification, counter-transference.

I would be happy if we went deeper into the meanings of her play. I would like to get tips on how to participate more actively in her play in order to achieve specific therapeutic goals.

Shlomo: We will discuss this case and other cases in our future meetings, and in doing so will expand the range of theoretical concepts and the tools available to us. I am impressed by your insights. See you in our next meeting.

Summary of chapter 1

In this chapter, my approach to play therapy is introduced. It has the following attributes: It is integrative – play therapy is not informed by a single theory (psychoanalytic, cognitive-behavioral, systemic, etc.) but by a synthesis of many theories. Individual, family and group play therapy can be conducted simultaneously. No specialized theoretical orientations or methods are used with different kinds of difficulties and syndromes. Suitable methods and techniques can be used with any kind of presenting difficulties. The choice of therapeutic vehicles is governed by a deep understanding of the case, not just by attempting to remove the external symptoms. Such understanding is achieved by a multi-systemic diagnosis. The therapist is not just a reflecting or interpreting observer of the clients' play. He is an active participant in the individual, group or family spontaneous play. As an active participant, he is an equal partner and a co-creator of the clients' play. This has many advantages: As one who has been admitted to the clients' play, the therapist is not perceived as a prying observer of the clients' intimate play, nor as an unwanted intruder. The partnership in the play allows the therapist great flexibility and provides him with an endless range of verbal and non-verbal therapeutic means.

Assignments

Describe in detail how you would join Rusella's play as described by Lailah in Session 1.1. What play moves would you make to achieve specific goals?

A classified list of publications

Non-directive and directive play-therapeutic models

Ariel, S., (1992). *Strategic family play therapy*. Chichester, UK: Wiley.

Baggerly, J.N., Ray, D.C. and Bratton, S.C., eds. (2010). *Child-centered play therapy research: The evidence base for effective practice*. Hoboken, NJ: Wiley.

Mullen, J.A. and Ickli, J. (2014). *Child-centered play therapy workbook: A self-directed guide for professionals*. Champaign, IL: Research Press Publishers.

Ryan, V. and Kate Wilson, K. (2000). *Case studies in non-directive play therapy*. Philadelphia, PA: Jessica Kingsley.

Schaefer, Ch.E., ed. (2011). *Foundations of play therapy: Second edition*. Hoboken, NJ: Wiley.

Integrative play therapy models

Ariel, S. (2018). *Multi-dimensional therapy with families, children and adults: The Diamond Model*. London, UK: Routledge.

Drewes, A. (2017). *Prescriptive integrative play therapy*. Washington, DC: American Psychological Association.

Drewes, A., Bratton, S.C. and Schaefer, Ch.E., eds. (2011). *Integrative play therapy*. Hoboken, NJ: Wiley.

Chapter 2
Appraising the current state of the art

The field of play therapy has made a great leap forward in recent years. Almost every major theoretical model in the various areas of psychotherapy has been expanded to include play therapy. Numerous new play-therapeutic concepts, methods and techniques have been made available to clinicians. Specialized play-therapeutic procedures for treating specific types of syndromes have been developed. Attempts to blend and integrate different play therapy models, e.g. dynamic and cognitive-behavioral, have been made. Interdisciplinary research has been done to establish the validity and efficacy of various play therapy models and techniques. A very large number of books and articles on play therapy have been published. Local and international play therapy professional organizations have been established. Play therapy courses, workshops and training programs are offered by many academic and professional institutes.

When I examine and contemplate about all this wealth, I am impressed and excited, but also feel that something is missing – conceptual clarity. The need to have a clearer view of the conceptual landscape of the play therapy field motivated me to try and clear the mental fog that disturbs this view. A great part of my academic work has been devoted to explicating vague or ambiguous concepts. The notion of *explication* was defined by the philosopher Rudolph Carnap as follows,

> Explication is the task of making more exact a vague or not quite exact concept used in everyday life or in an earlier stage of scientific or logical development, or rather by replacing it by a newly constructed, more exact concept.
> (Carnap, 1950, pp. 8–9)

Explication in Carnap's sense does not necessarily require adherence to the original contexts in which the concept to be explicated has been used.

Here are concepts that, in my view, must be explicated in order to place the play therapy field on a more solid foundation:

What is *play*?

To judge the validity of the various assumptions and empirical studies concerning the therapeutic powers of play and the efficacy of play therapy, the concept *play* must be explicated. Trezza et al. (2010) assert that play releases, through the brain's limbic system, "happy chemicals", associated with enjoyable experiences and positive emotions. When I read this statement, I asked myself, "What do they mean by *play*? What kind of play? What exactly in what they call *play* is responsible for those blissful experiences?"

In natural language, concepts are not defined with scientific precision. The word "play" in English refers to all sorts of phenomena that do not have much in common, although they somehow feel akin. The English language distinguishes between *play* and *game*. Some other languages use the same word for these seemingly different entities. We say that American football is "played by two teams of eleven players". This activity is so violent and dangerous that the players must wear a helmet with metal bars to protect their head and faces and protective pads, not to mention the fact that it is a very big business. Would you include this kind of activity under the same title as a little girl pretending to be a fairy?

There are terms in natural language and in professional literature that relate to different types of play and games: Rough and tumble play, practice play (Piaget, 1962), pretend or make-believe play, sociodramatic play, board games, games with rules (Piaget, 1962), competitive games, etc. What do all these have in common?

In the play therapy literature, there is a place of honor for the kind of individual or social play called *pretend play*, *make-believe play*, *thematic play*, etc. I like the term *make-believe play* best. I do not believe that the cover terms *play* or *game*, which relate to the entire range of phenomena detailed above, can be explicated by a single definition. I do believe however that the concept *make-believe play* can be explicated by an exact formal definition. Various attempts have been made to propose such a definition. The most famous among them is Winnicott's (1971) definition of (make-believe) play as something that happens in the interface between our inner world and external reality, taking place neither strictly in our imagination, nor in the truly external world. Although this definition makes intuitive sense, to my mind it is still too vague. In Chapter 8, a fully explicit, exact formal definition of the concept of make-believe play is presented. This definition makes it possible to distinguish in a clear-cut manner between make-believe play and other superficially similar phenomena, such as other kinds of play, fantasy, imitation and so forth. It has far-reaching implications with respect to understanding the therapeutic applications of this kind of play.

What is *play therapy*?

Play therapy is defined in the website of the North American Association of Play Therapy as "the systematic use of a theoretical model to establish an interpersonal process wherein trained play therapists use the therapeutic powers of play to help clients prevent or resolve psychosocial difficulties and achieve optimal growth and development". I have no quarrel with this definition, but I think it should be clarified. There are some conditions that a theoretical model must meet if it is to serve as a reliable guide for play-therapeutic work:

(a) The model must explain the difficulties that require treatment, expose their root causes, pinpoint their sources. A mechanic will not start repairing a vehicle before he identifies the source of the problem. A doctor will not perform surgery and prescribe drugs before having diagnosed the disease.
(b) The model must expose all the causal agents that influence the difficulties, not just some of them. A mechanic who finds a problem with the engine but ignores a problem in the electrical system will not be able to fix the vehicle. This analogy applies to a doctor too.
(c) The model must include suitable healing tools and procedures that tackle effectively all the previously identified sources of the difficulties.

I don't know of any model of play therapy that meets all three of these conditions. A model that does fulfill all three of them must address the multiple genetic, developmental, cultural and environmental factors involved in psychopathology and other kinds of difficulties brought to therapy. It should acknowledge the fact that some children lack the ability to play at all or the ability to activate the therapeutic powers of play. It must include precautions against the danger that the client be re-traumatized by his or her play.

In order to know what play therapy is and what it is not, one must know first, as required above, what play is and what it is not. The play therapy literature abounds with methods in which what is taken to be play is just a teaching aid, facilitating the learning of some ideas and skills by illustrating them. Some procedures considered play therapy are structured, directive, protocolled activities, using cards or board games. Such procedures obey strict rules and do not leave much room for imagination, creativity or spontaneous therapeutic processes. There are numerous ingenious fun-filled techniques, engaging clients in therapeutically useful activities. No doubt these are very serviceable, but should they be considered play-therapeutic? In many play therapy publications, the boundaries between play therapy, creative arts therapy, drama therapy, movement therapy, bibliotherapy, etc., are not clearly delineated. I am not a purist. I don't think the concept of play therapy should necessarily be delimited to therapeutic processes driven by spontaneous play, but I believe this field will benefit from a definition of its essence and boundaries.

In this book I chose to focus on play therapy in which the therapist is an active participant in the clients' spontaneous play, especially make-believe play. Free, spontaneous play includes storytelling, drama, art, movement, music and various other expressive media.

Play as a language

The assertion that play is a language appears repeatedly in the play therapy literature. Indeed, play, especially make-believe play, is a language in the wide sense of the term, a semiotic system with its own vocabulary, grammar, syntax, semantics and pragmatics (i.e. its uses in contexts). It is important for a play therapist to possess the conceptual and technical tools for analyzing the play language of the clients and to formulate its rules. These tools will enable the therapist to decipher the play, its overt and covert meanings and functions, and communicate with the players in their own play language. Such tools are introduced in Chapters 4–7.

Some preconceived ideas about the nature of play as a language have put down roots among many play therapists. Gary Landreth's often cited maxim, "Toys are the children's words and play is their language," (2002, p. 303) is, to my mind, misleading. It disregards the fact that very often make-believe play is purely verbal, or both verbal and non-verbal. It does not consider the fact that the means of make-believe play are not just toys but any tangible entities – pieces of paper, sounds, the player's body, etc. It misses the fact that, unlike words, any tangible entity can be assigned a potentially infinite number of meanings. Such tangible entities are not like words but more like the speech sounds of language. They are the raw materials of the play.

Another statement often found in the play therapy literature is that verbal therapy does not suit young children because their command of language and their verbal meta-cognition capacity are still rather limited. That is why play is the preferable medium for child therapy. This statement implies that play is non-verbal and does not allow for meta-cognition. This is incorrect. Many children as young as four or five often use rich verbal language in their play. They are quite sophisticated in their use of language. Meta-cognition is an inherent property of make-believe play because children distinguish between play and non-play and often comment about the contents of their own play. Here is a fragment from an interactional make-believe play of a 4.6-year-old girl, Shir, where she is telling me:

> Let's play as if I see a beggar in the street and give him money but I don't show him that I feel sorry for him because I really do feel sorry for him, but I don't want to show it to him, so he will not be offended. You'll be the beggar and I'll be the other Shir, OK?

Proliferation of models and attempts at integration

The fertile ground of the field of play has produced scores of models, each presented as different and unique. Most of these have extended existing models to host play therapy: Psychoanalytic play therapy, Jungian play therapy, Adlerian play therapy, Gestalt play therapy, cognitive-behavioral play therapy, and so forth. Most of these models share at least some basic assumptions, concepts, methods and techniques, disguised in different terminologies.

It is no wonder that many attempts have been made to integrate or blend different models. However, to the best of my knowledge there have been no attempts to create a theoretical and applicational integration of the entire play therapy field. Most attempts at integration have combined no more than two models:

Psychodynamic and cognitive-behavioral, filial therapy and attachment-based therapy, eco-systemic therapy and theraplay, etc. In most cases, the integration has been done with reference to a specific type of syndrome. I have not found any attempt to create a theoretical integration in the full sense of the word, that is, synthesizing two or more theoretical models into a single new model. (See Drewes, 2009; Drewes, Bratton and Schaefer, 2011.)

In some cases, it has been proposed to approach a case by drawing on two different theoretical models, with the original models remaining intact. In other cases, the approach adopted has been what is termed *assimilative integration*, that is, working in the framework of one model but borrowing techniques from other models, if this is considered beneficial for the therapy. Another approach has been *technical eclecticism*, that is, borrowing techniques from multiple sources without adopting the conceptual worlds in which these techniques had been created. (See Stricker and Gold, 2013.)

In my view, this multiplicity of partial integrations still leaves the field too fragmented. Take for instance Case 1.1 (Rusella) and the ensuing discussion in the interdisciplinary seminar. Obviously, the participants were somewhat overwhelmed, confused and disoriented by the complexity of the case (which is not different from that of any other case), and by the multiplicity of theoretical concepts and possible approaches. Trainees, as well as experienced therapists, would benefit if they had at their disposal a full, rather than partial integrative theoretical model. Such a model is introduced in this book. It does not pretend to encompass the entire field, but it is comprehensive enough to serve as a road map that facilitates orientation in most cases brought to therapy. I call this model the Diamond Model, because, like a diamond, it is multi-faceted and lucid. Integrative play therapy is subsumed under the Diamond Model.

The Diamond Model is outlined in Chapter 3. It is introduced more fully in Ariel (2018).

Summary of chapter 2

This chapter presents a brief appraisal of the current state of the art of play therapy. Despite the dramatic growth of the field, some key concepts are still rather vague and ambiguous. Adopting the philosopher Rudolf Carnap's concept of *explication*, an attempt is presented to disambiguate the very concepts *play* and *play therapy*. It is stated that one of the kinds of play, *make-believe play*, can and will be defined rigorously. Key therapeutic properties of play can be derived from this definition. It is asserted that the concept of *play therapy* is over-inclusive. It is argued that every model of play therapy should provide a full explanation of each case and supply all the means for tackling all the relevant aspects of the case. It is stated that play may be viewed and analyzed as a language, a semiotic system. Some misconceptions are pointed out, e.g. that play therapy, being non-verbal, suits young children because they are not yet verbally sophisticated and lack meta-cognition ability. Finally, it is argued that despite some attempts at integration, the field of play therapy is still too fragmented theoretically and methodologically. The work presented in this book constitutes an attempt at a full comprehensive integration of this field.

> ### Assignments
> 1. Tell the differences between play and games, and between different kinds of play and games.
> 2. In what senses is play a language?
> 3. Give three examples of verbal make-believe play and three examples of meta-cognition in make-believe play.
> 4. Which psychotherapy models should be integrated into a single comprehensive model in order to address all the aspects of Case 1.1 (Rusella)?

A classified list of publications

Explication

Carnap, R. (1950). *Logical foundations of probability*. London, UK: Routledge and Kegan Paul.

Definitions of the concept play

Ariel, S. (2002). *Children's imaginative play: A visit to Wonderland*. Westport, CT: Praeger.
Bateson, G. (1956). The message 'this is play'. In: Schaffner, B., ed. *Group processes: Transactions of the second conference*. New York, NY: Josiah Macy, Jr. Foundation, pp.145–242.
Piaget, J. (1962). *Play, dreams and imitation in childhood*. New York, NY: Norton.
Winnicott, D. (1971). *Playing and Reality*. London, UK: Tavistock.

Definitions of the concept play therapy

Schaefer, Ch. and Drewes, A.A., eds. (2013). *The therapeutic powers of play: 20 core agents of change, 2nd edition*. Hoboken, NJ: Wiley.
Schaefer, Ch. and Kaduson, H.G. (1994). *The quotable play therapist: 238 of the all-time best quotes on play and play therapy*. Northvale, NJ: Jason Aronson.

The pleasure of playing

Trezza V., Baarendse P.J.J. and Vanderschuren L.J.M.J. (2010). The pleasures of play: Pharmacological insights into social reward mechanisms. *Trends in Pharmacological Science* 31, pp.463–469.

Play as a language

Ariel, S. (2002). *Children's imaginative play: A visit to Wonderland*. Westport, CT: Praeger.
Bruner, J. (1983). Play, thought and language. *Peabody Journal of Education* 60 (3), pp.60–69.
Landreth, G.L. (2002). *Play therapy: The art of relationship*. UK: Routledge.

Psychotherapy integration and integrative play therapy

Ariel, S. (2018). *Multi-dimensional therapy with families, children and adults: The Diamond Model*. London, UK: Routledge.
Drewes, A.A. (2009). *Blending play therapy with cognitive behavioral therapy: Evidence-based and other effective treatments and techniques*. Hoboken, NJ: Wiley.
Drewes, A.A., Bratton, S.C. and Schaefer, Ch., eds. (2011). *Integrative play therapy*. Hoboken, NJ: Wiley.
Stricker, G. and Gold. J., eds. (2013). *A casebook of psychotherapy integration*. Washington, DC: American Psychological Association.

Chapter 3

The Diamond Model

The discussion of Case 1.1 (Rusella) in the (fictitious) interdisciplinary seminar in Chapter 1 is typical of such discussions. There is no such thing as a simple case, and Rusella's case is no exception. The participants found the case complex and not easy to decipher. They had a lot to say and used quite a few theoretical concepts from different models, but it was difficult for them to put everything together and find a clear and focused direction for understanding the case and deciding on the right therapy. One of the reasons why I have developed the Diamond Model is to reduce the typical sense of confusion and of being overwhelmed, which almost inevitably accompanies any attempt to understand a case and know how to approach it. The Diamond Model is designed, in a sense, to simplify our attempts to understand a case and treat it. The Diamond Model is introduced in Ariel (2018). Here is a brief summary of its main elements:

The Diamond Model is multi-systemic

Every case brought to therapy, whatever the presenting difficulties, is multi-determined, a product of a dynamic interaction between factors (I prefer the term *programs*) belonging to many different internal and external subsystems. Therefore, the Diamond Model is multi-systemic.

The internal subsystems (within the individual) are:

the body (the brain and the nervous system, the genetic, anatomic and physiological subsystems);
the cognitive and psychomotor subsystems;
conscious or unconscious emotional concerns, emotional conflicts and emotional defenses;
the individual and social personality (self and body images and concepts, object relations, self and body boundaries, attachment, egocentricity and narcissism vs. empathy and prosocial attitude, reality testing, self-control, psychosexual development, moral development);
the internalized culture.

The external subsystems are:

significant life events;
the family and other social systems;
the ecosystems (the human and nonhuman environment at large).

Each of the subsystems and all of them can be looked at *synchronically* (a cross section at a time, usually the beginning of therapy) or *diachronically* (from the past to the present, development through time). Both the external subsystems and the internal subsystems keep changing and developing. The diagnostic assessment and the therapy should consider such changes and developments. It is also important to have a *developmental profile* of each client, across all the internal systems that are relevant to the case.

In designing and carrying out the therapy, all the relevant programs and their interrelations must be considered. Ignoring relevant programs found in any of the subsystems can result in understanding the case incorrectly and choosing an ineffective or even harmful therapeutic strategy.

Developmental profiles

Development on all the developmental lines, in any of the internal subsystems, advances through the following dimensions: growth, internalization, complexity, coordination and integration, differentiation, depth of processing, concreteness vs., abstraction, flexibility, constancy and stability, objectivity, monitoring and control, socialization.

Not all the dimensions are relevant to every line, however.

An accurate developmental profile can be obtained by formal standardized tests. A therapist who lacks expertise in administering such tests can still estimate clients' developmental profiles by observations and interviews. Observing spontaneous play can provide rich information about the players' level of development in all areas. Methods of obtaining such information from observed play are presented in Chapters 4–7.

Syndromes such as internalized disorders (e.g. anxiety, depression, inhibitions), externalizing disorders (e.g. conduct disorders), post-traumatic stress disorder, etc., can be conceptualized as products of below-age-level development on various dimensions in various subsystems, due to genetic causes, environmental factors, lacunae, fixation, regression, splitting and dissociation, emotion-dysregulation, inadequate defenses related to specific emotions and faulty ("bugged", see below) information-processing programs. Therapy in general and play therapy in particular should therefore aim at restoring emotion balance, weakening harmful defenses, removing or weakening bugs in information-processing programs and resuming the capacity for normal development.

A uniform, explicit theoretical language

Another trait that meets the challenge posed by complex, confusing cases is common language. The whole discourse in the Diamond Model can be formulated in a single uniform, accurate, formal language purported to be universally applicable. The choice of language is not arbitrary but empirically based. The language employed in the Diamond Model consists of three sub-languages: The sub-language of *semiotics*, (the science of signs and symbols), the sublanguage of *information-processing* and the sub-language of *cybernetics*, (the science of systems of regulation and control, using concepts such as *homeostasis, corrective feedback* and *feed-forward*).

All the internal and external subsystems listed above can be reformulated in the vocabulary and grammar of these three sub-languages. Rusella's choice to speak in a babyish voice can be analyzed and reformulated in these three sub-languages. In the semiotic language it can be said that talking in a babyish voice has meaning and communicative functions. It signifies a baby who still does not know how to speak clearly. It enables Rusella to say whatever comes to her mind without censorship, by making herself unintelligible. In information-processing terms, the babyish talk can be formulated as an information-processing program of which the input is abusive behavior on the side of her peers and mother and the output is infantile speech. The internal processing is the interpretation of the input as responses to Rusella's age and physical and cognitive limitations.

In the cybernetic language, the concept of *homeostasis* refers to the tendency of organisms to auto-regulate and maintain their internal environment in a stable, harmonious, balanced state, a state of equilibrium. For example, heart rate is coordinated with the body's intake of oxygen. When the body exerts more effort, it needs more oxygen, so the heart rate increases, to get more oxygen. When the body rests, the heart rate decreases. Any deviation from the desired homeostasis is corrected by these regulative processes. If something goes wrong in this regulative mechanism, *feed-forward* can happen instead of corrective feedback. For instance, when the body invests less effort and no longer needs a large amount of oxygen, the deviation from the homeostatic, balanced state is nevertheless amplified unabated. The heart rate increases without stopping.

These cybernetic terms are applicable to information-processing programs in each and all the internal and external subsystems. For example, a girl who is worried about her weight gain will be weighed over and over again. She will look at herself in the mirror and listen to responses from her friends. This corrective feedback will convince her that her weight has not risen, and she will calm down. The input and the internal processing will be balanced, will be in a homeostatic state. But all these corrective feedbacks will not convince an anorexic girl, and will only encourage her to eat less.

These sub-languages are introduced in more detail in Ariel (1992, 1999, 2002 and 2018).

A central explanatory principle – simplicity

A third trait of the Diamond Model that meets the challenge posed by complex, confusing cases is applying one central principle for explaining the etiology of each case and the processes of spontaneous and therapeutic change. The key concept in this explanatory format is *simplicity*. In the Diamond Model, well-functioning programs are defined as *programs that are cybernetically sound*, programs that can mobilize corrective feedback and restore deviations from the homeostatic balance of the subsystem to which they belong. This concept applies to programs of any of the internal or external subsystems. Loss of the previous simplicity of external and internal subsystems in times of change and crisis, and abortive attempts to restore simplicity, throw the subsystems off-balance, causing emotion dysregulation, loss of homeostasis and inability to mobilize corrective feedback. The purpose of therapy is to create a new simplicity.

Take for instance a girl whose father began to sexually abuse her when she reached adolescence. Before that, her relationship with her father was optimally simple. She knew what to expect from her father's behavior toward her in most situations and was able to correctly interpret his physical expressions of affection. Then, the previous simplicity was lost. Her father began to behave toward her in a way she had never known before. At first it was hard for her to decide whether his new way of touching her was an expression of affection or sexual exploitation. She began to feel shame, fear and anger and did not know how to react.

The same notion, simplicity, is also the criterion for testing the relative validity of the interpretations given to cases. The most valid *idiographic theory* (a theory applying to a single case) is the simplest one.

There are programs that have never been optimally simple in the above sense. Such programs are found, for example, in children whose information-processing capacities in any of the internal subsystems are genetically impaired, or in interpersonal subsystems, e.g. the parental one, that have been dysfunctional right from the very beginning. It would be wrong, however, to assume that such programs are hopelessly dysfunctional. In most cases, the right therapeutic interventions can help them become simpler and improve their functioning.

Each program and each set of programs in any internal or external subsystem is optimally simple and cybernetically sound if it can process all the information that is relevant to adequate functioning in a consistent and correct manner. In more detail, a program or a set of programs is optimally simple if it is *comprehensive, parsimonious, consistent* and *plausible*.

Comprehensiveness: The programs can take in, retrieve from memory, process and produce as output all the information needed for a subsystem to function adequately and maintain a homeostatic, balanced state.

Parsimony: The program or set of programs can take in, retrieve, processes and produce as output only information that is relevant to good functioning.

Consistency: The program or set of programs does not include self-contradictions.

Plausibility: The program or set of programs interprets the information correctly and makes correct predictions as to the results of the output produced.

Consider for instance a person who lives in a closed ethnically and culturally uniform religious community, e.g. an Ultra-Orthodox Jewish community. His interpersonal programs are comprehensive. He knows how to process all the information needed for adequate interpersonal functioning in his social environment. His interpersonal programs are parsimonious. He does not need to process irrelevant information such as thinking about what style of clothing to adopt. His programs are consistent. His culinary programs are consistent. He always eats only kosher food. His programs are plausible. He knows how to correctly interpret, for instance, being ignored by a man mumbling a prayer.

In the Diamond Model, programs that lack comprehensiveness, parsimony, consistency or plausibility are termed *bugged programs*. The *bugs* were given, respectively, the following mnemonic names:

Lack of comprehensiveness: *Horse blinders*.
Lack of parsimony: *Fifth wheel*.
Lack of consistency: *Flip-flop*.
Lack of plausibility: *Non-sense*.

The etiology of difficulties referred to therapy can be explained in many cases as resulting from bugs that had invaded programs in any subsystem. In the history of the case, programs become bugged, characteristically, in periods of drastic change and crisis, in which the previous optimally simple programs have lost their simplicity, e.g. in circumstances of illness or death in the family, loss of a job, war or culture change.

In such periods, the previous programs lose their comprehensiveness. They encounter information they had not been equipped to take in and process (*horse blinders*). The adolescent girl whose father began to abuse her sexually had not experienced such parental behavior in her previous parent–daughter programs.

In such a situation, the old programs also lose their parsimony. The old codes of behavior are no longer relevant. They become redundant (*fifth wheel*). The innocent physical expressions of affection on the part of the father of the adolescent girl were no longer relevant to their changed relationship.

In periods of change and crisis the previous programs often lose their consistency (*flip-flop*). They can no longer process the new information in a consistent manner. The adolescent girl could no longer give a consistent interpretation to her father's new way of touching her.

In such periods, the previous programs lose their plausibility (*non-sense*). They have no longer the required means to interpret the new information correctly or to make correct predictions. The adolescent girl no longer knew how to interpret her father's physical advances.

The loss of simplicity in this sense often throws the person's cognitive-emotion subsystems off-balance. This usually happens if the change or crisis is sudden or overwhelming. In cybernetic terms, the arousal of emotions such as fear, anxiety, sadness or anger cannot be stopped and re-balanced by corrective feedback.

Instead, feed-forward processes are set into operation. The arousal of unpleasant emotions increases unabated and the output becomes more and more dysfunctional. The emotion dysregulation and the dysfunctional output make it extremely difficult to adapt to the new circumstances by making the necessary adjustments in the previous programs.

A characteristic dysfunctional defensive "solution" adopted in such situations is *restoring the lost simplicity partially*: Consistency is maintained at the cost of comprehensiveness, parsimony and plausibility, in other words, the relevant programs are not infected with flip-flop but are infected with horse blinders, fifth wheel and non-sense. Comprehensiveness is preserved at the cost of parsimony, consistency and plausibility, in other words, the relevant programs are not infected with horse blinders but are infected with fifth wheel, flip-flop and non-sense, and so forth. The abused adolescent girl attempts to re-balance the off-balanced emotions related to the loss of simplicity of her relationship with her father by preserving consistency at the cost of comprehensiveness, parsimony and plausibility. For instance, she can blame herself entirely for her father's abuse, ignoring his own guilt (non-sense and horse blinders). Or she can co-operate with her father's abuse, subconsciously pretending that nothing has changed in their previous relationship (non-sense, horse blinders and fifth wheel). She can adopt another "solution", preserving comprehensiveness and plausibility at the cost of consistency. She will understand that her father's abusive behavior is totally wrong. At the same time, she will not ignore the positive sides in his personality. She will fluctuate between co-operating with him and "understanding" him on the one hand, and rejecting and blaming him on the other hand. All these strategies are dysfunctional. They set into operation deviation-amplifying feed-forward processes. If she blames herself, she will feel more and more guilty, hate herself and will not do anything to stop the abuse. If she co-operates with her father's abuse, she will not really feel better and will not stop her father's aggression. If she reacts inconsistently, her mental confusion and stress will be augmented and, again, she will give her father a double message that would not help him contend with his own crime.

The dysfunction in such situations can start in one or two programs and spread to more and more programs in various subsystems, like cancer.

Effective therapy therefore requires removing or weakening the bugs. Since what energizes the bugs are emotions that got off-balance, the successful removal of the bugs requires restoring emotional balance. The therapy should concentrate first on emotion-balancing, using suitable techniques, and then on removing the bugs by what I term *bug-busters*.

As noted above, the diagnostic assessment and therapy should take into account the developmental profile of the clients. Bug-busters can promote learning and development processes too. All these can be achieved by play therapy. Emotion-balancing play techniques, play bug-busters and ways of promoting learning and development by play are introduced in Chapters 8–11 and 15–17.

Understanding change mechanisms – technical eclecticism

What makes bug-busters work? Technical eclecticism is one of the pillars of the psychotherapy integration movement. I have surveyed many therapeutic models and traditional healing practices and found out that the techniques they employ can be classified under a limited number of types of change-mechanisms. If a therapist understands the change-mechanism that makes a technique work, he/she can borrow the right technique for the task in hand (restoring emotion-balance, removing bugs and promoting change and development), or make up his/her own techniques that activate these change-mechanisms.

The types of change-mechanisms are: working through the body – changing body functions; enhancing alertness, attention and concentration; influence and suggestion; expression and catharsis; positive reinforcement and support; habituation; concretization; influencing information-processing. (See Ariel, 2018, Chapter 9.)

One of the most important recent developments in the field of play therapy has been the attempt to identify and define the therapeutic powers of play, in other words, the types of change mechanisms inherent in play. (See Schaefer and Drewes, 2013.) The types of change mechanisms listed above are applicable to play therapy and are consistent with the categories of therapeutic powers of play documented in the publication referred to above. A re-examination of the therapeutic powers of play discussed in the literature is presented in detail in Chapter 12.

Interdisciplinary seminar

Here is another session with Lailah (a clinical psychologist), Daniel (a social worker), Anna (a creative arts therapist) and Ethan (a school psychologist).

Shlomo: Let's now examine the onset of bugs from a diachronic perspective. Here is a brief summary of the history of a case. The family was treated in the framework of the local social services for six years. I was the case manager.

Case 3.1 Max
Max, 12, said he wanted to die, because his mother did not love him and did not want him. She preferred his nine-year-old brother Danny, and Max felt she would have gotten rid of him gladly if only she had a choice. He said he missed his late father, who was the only one who really loved him and cared for him.

Danny claimed that Max was harassing him, beating him, calling him names and taking his things, without any provocation on his part. Their mother, Sabina, insisted that she loved both her sons equally and did not discriminate against either of them. She said she was a dedicated mother. Her sons were her whole life. Max was constantly putting her love to the test, she said. He would demand that she cook him the food he likes, and then would refuse to eat it, accusing her of deliberately preparing him spoiled food. He would make her buy him things he didn't need, and so on.

Six years earlier, Sabina had contacted the social services, seeking couple's therapy. She arrived with her husband, Alex. She claimed that he had forced her to sell an apartment she had inherited from her parents to finance his failing business. He claimed that the business was growing and developing and eventually would bring great profits. She should be less impatient and distrustful. She said he was insulting her, calling her stupid, fat and ugly. He said she was driving him crazy, causing him to freak out. She said he took over the older son, Max, appropriating him as if she wasn't his mother and inciting him against her. He said she didn't understand the boy and was constantly hurting his feelings.

Alex did not show up for the next session and did not return to therapy. It took Sabina years to gather courage and demand divorce. She was afraid of Alex. She saw him as vengeful and violent.

On the day of their divorce, Alex kidnapped Max and disappeared. Max did not show up in school and did not contact Sabina. She decided not to involve the police. She did her own detective work and managed to find the hideout in a slum part of the city where Alex held Max. She hid until she saw that Alex was leaving the house, and then went into the apartment. Max looked bad, neglected and scared. He did not let her touch him and refused to come back home with her. Sabina decided not to involve the authorities, so as not to exacerbate Max's trauma. When Alex was not home, she would bring Max food, clothing and other necessities. She hoped to persuade him gradually to return home.

A few months later she learned that Alex died of cardiac arrest, but she suspected he had committed suicide. Max returned home.

Anna: Depressing. I feel so sorry for Max.
Shlomo: Maybe it would be an anti-climax to analyze this dramatic true story with the analytical tools of the Diamond Model, but let's try. I'd like us to focus on the loss of simplicity (comprehensiveness, parsimony, consistency and plausibility) in stressful periods of extreme change and crisis and on bug-producing attempts to restore simplicity partially.
Ethan: It seems that the entire life of this family had been characterized by extreme stress, but the main crisis periods were the divorce and the kidnapping of Max by his father Alex, the latter's death and Max's return to Sabina's home.
Lailah: Before the divorce and the abduction, the relationship between Alex and Sabina was terrible. They couldn't agree on anything and he would insult her and take over Max. Is it true to say that the family system had been optimally simple then? Was it plausible?
Daniel: Max wasn't really abducted. He left with his father on his own accord.
Ethan: But he was a minor!
Shlomo: One should distinguish between *plausible* and *reasonable*. Plausibility means correct interpretations of the input and the memory materials, and correct predictions.

Anna: Did Alex and Sabina correctly interpret each other?
Daniel: As for his business, it is difficult to judge. Maybe the business really had a chance of succeeding. Maybe she was impatient.
Ethan: Maybe she really was fat and ugly and stupid? Don't take me seriously. (Only the boys are laughing.)
Anna: Apparently, she understood correctly his appropriation of Max, but his accusations that she did not understand Max and hurt his feelings were probably unfounded.
Ethan: Unfounded, bugged with non-sense and perhaps also horse blinders.
Lailah: We lack data, especially about how the children perceived the situation. Anyway, I don't think the relationship between Alex and Sabina was inconsistent, so there was no flip-flop bug there. It is also hard for me to judge whether there was also a lack of relevance, a fifth wheel.
Ethan: According to family systems theory, the conflict with respect to Max was not relevant to the real problems in the relationship between Alex and Sabina. Max was triangulated.
Anna: So, what was the real conflict about?
Ethan: About money, exploitation, lack of love and friendship.
Shlomo: There is much more to say about what happened before the kidnapping or whatever we call it. As for the business for instance, we see a lack of comprehensiveness, horse blinders, on both sides. Alex ignored the fact that Sabina had agreed to sell the apartment not willingly but under pressure, that she really feared the money would be lost. Sabina did not consider Alex's need to succeed, to prove himself and to support his family. We lack data, but it is reasonable to assume that the turning point in their relationship was the sale of the apartment.

Let's skip to Max's return home after his father's death.

Daniel: Clearly, Max wore enormous horse blinders and was infected with non-sense.
Lailah: All his life he had been brainwashed by his father.
Anna: Perhaps he felt unconsciously that reuniting with his mother and brother would be a betrayal of his father's memory. Since he had been kidnapped, his life was a trauma on top of a trauma on top of a trauma.
Shlomo: Let's look at his faulty processing of the input received from his mother and brother and the data retrieved from memory in terms of his attempt to restore the lost simplicity partially.
(Silence.)
Ethan:Tell us. We are not used to work with these concepts.
Shlomo: OK. I think he unconsciously maintained consistency at the expense of comprehensiveness, plausibility and parsimony. In other words, his proxmity-control programs with respect to Sabina and Danny were infected with horse blinders, non-sense and fifth wheel, but not with flip-flop. The contradiction

between his faith that his father had all his life protected him from his mother, loved him wholeheartedly and cared for him on the one hand, and the recognition that his father really had abused him and robbed him of his loving and caring mother on the other hand, was emotionally intolerable.

Daniel: He had to choose between his mother and his father as primary attachment figures.

Shlomo: Yes. So, he consistently kept within himself the internalized image of his father, including the latter's attitude toward his mother, which was no longer relevant to his current life (fifth wheel). He ignored all the data that could refute this stereotypical view of his mother and misinterpreted her behavior toward him (horse blinders and non-sense). In cybernetic terms, these bugs prevented him from mobilizing corrective feedback, which could allow him to use all the relevant information and interpret the input correctly, and in this way fully restore his lost simplicity. His responses (output) toward Sabina and Danny just invited counter-responses that "proved" him right. The vicious circle created in this way brought about feed-forward instead of corrective feedback, that is, an increasingly amplified deviation for the harmonious homeostasis between the mutual proximity-control programs of Sabina, Max and Danny.

Lailah: I don't believe I will be ever able to formulate it in this way.

Shlomo: Don't worry, you will.

Anna: How can we break this vicious circle?

Shlomo: We'll have to find ways to help Max, Sabina and Danny balance the dysregulated emotions that prevent the bugs from being weakened or disappearing and use various techniques that I term *bug-busters*.

Anna: Can this be achieved by play therapy?

Shlomo: Yes, we can help the family activate the emotion-balancing mechanism of play and help them utilize what I term *play bug-busters*. We'll discuss and illustrate these in our coming meetings. These concepts need to be operationalized. At this stage let us consider them as broad categories, of which the applicability to the case data will be partly intuitive.

Daniel: Let me try to apply some of these categories to Max. His level of development in the subsystem of attachment to a mother figure was low.

Shlomo: In what parameters?

Daniel: (Scanning the list of parameters) I think internalization, differentiation, and depth of processing. He didn't internalize the positive aspects of his mother's behavior toward him and did not differentiate between different aspects of his mother's behavior. He processed his mother's input on a very superficial processing level.

Ethan: Also, complexity. His internalized mother image was very simplistic.

Lailah: It seems to me also that his level of development was low also in the areas of egocentricity and narcissism vs. empathy, pro-social attitude and reality testing. The relevant parameters are socialization and objectivity.

Shlomo: Considering that I did not define all of these concepts for you fully and accurately, your analysis is not bad at all. However, it is important to understand whether these really reflect a low level of development or just defenses. This distinction is important for our diagnostic evaluation and for predicting what will work in therapy and what will not.

Summary of chapter 3

This chapter is devoted to a brief presentation of the Diamond Model, an integrative model that is supposed to guide and simplify the whole diagnostic and therapeutic work. This model has the following traits: It is multi-systemic. Every case is a product of a dynamic interaction of programs belonging to many subsystems within the person (genetic, anatomic, physiological, psychomotor, cognitive, emotional, personality-developmental and cultural) and outside the person (life events, family and other social systems, ecology). The subsystems can be looked at synchronically or diachronically. Each of the internal programs develops along fixed parameters. The Diamond Model is a synthesis of concepts and methods drawn from multiple sources. It is linguistically uniform. The whole diagnostic and therapeutic discourse can be formulated in the same explicit theoretical languages – semiotics, information-processing and cybernetics. The etiology of each case is explained by the same principle of simplicity. Well-functioning programs in all the subsystems are optimally simple, that is, can process all and only the information needed for proper functioning in consistent and plausible manners. In other words, they are comprehensive, parsimonious, consistent and plausible. Programs can lose their simplicity in periods of drastic change and crisis, in which the persons' emotions get off-balance. They become infected with *bugs* – horse blinders (lack of comprehensiveness), fifth-wheel (lack of parsimony), flip-flop (lack of consistency) and non-sense (lack of plausibility). A typical dysfunctional strategy used in such situations is restoring simplicity partially (e.g. preserving consistency at the cost of comprehensiveness, plausibility and parsimony), leaving the bugs intact. The bugs prevent the programs from enlisting homeostasis-maintaining corrective feedback. The result is dysfunctional feed-forward, escalating deviation from the desired homeostasis. This can explain the formation of various psychological symptoms and other difficulties, as well as the occurrence of developmental disorders on the various parameters. Therapy in general and play therapy in particular should aim at removing or weakening the bugs, by restoring the balance of bugs-maintaining emotions that got off-balance, and by activating various "bug-busters" or "play bug-busters". Therapy should also aim at restoring the program's capacity of learning and development. (e) The choice or creation of bug-busters, emotion-balancing techniques and techniques promoting learning and development is subject to the principle of technical eclecticism. Any technique from any source can be employed if it can serve the above-mentioned purposes.

Assignments

1. Explain the following concepts, using your own words, and illustrate them with your own clinical examples or with examples drawn from the literature: subsystems within the individual and subsystems outside the individual; multi-systemic; semiotics; human information-processing; information-processing programs; cybernetics; homeostasis; corrective feedback; feed-forward; simplicity; comprehensiveness, parsimony, consistency and plausibility; loss of simplicity in periods of change and crisis; bugs; horse blinders, fifth wheel, flip-flop, non-sense; restoring simplicity partially; bug-busters; play bug-busters; technical eclecticism.
2. Attempt to apply the concepts of the Diamond Model to your own life history.
3. Analyze the following case, using the concepts of the Diamond Model:

Case 3.2 Kabr

Nine-year-old Kabr was diagnosed as ADHD. Two of his uncles on his father's side and one son of each also seemed to suffer from ADHD, although they have not been diagnosed as such. When Kabr started school, he couldn't concentrate in class and got confused in math and reading. This lowered his self-image. He used to feel ashamed, inferior, thought that his teachers, parents and peers looked down on him. His younger sister was better at school than him. In his culture, a son should be better than a daughter and this hurt his honor and self-respect even further. Because of all that he used to hide at home and would not go out to play with friends. This adversely affected his social development. He had an older brother who used to call him lazy and said he should be punished. In this culture an older brother has authority over a younger brother. His mother took his side but his father and uncles on the father's side (the ones who was also ADHD) agreed with his older brother. They were also afraid that he would drop out of school and become a delinquent like many kids in the neighborhood.

A classified list of publications

The Diamond Model

Ariel, S. (2018). *Multi-dimensional therapy with families, children and adults: The Diamond Model*. London, UK: Routledge.

Multi-systemic psychotherapy and psychotherapy integration

Brooks-Harris, J.E. (2008). *Integrative multitheoretical psychotherapy*. Boston, MA: Houghton-Mifflin.
Casonguay, L., Eubanks, C.F., Goldfried, M.R., Muran, J. Ch. and Lutz, W. (2015). Research on psychotherapy integration: Building on the past, looking for the future. *Psychotherapy Research*, 25(3), pp.365–382.
Norcross, J.C. and Goldfried, M.R., eds. (2005). *Handbook of psychotherapy integration*. Oxford, UK: Oxford University Press.
Wachtel, P.L. (1997). *Psychoanalysis, behavior therapy, and the relational world*. Washington, DC: American Psychological Association.

Explication, systematization and formalization

Bandler, R. and Grinder, J. (1975). *The structure of magic: A book about language and therapy*. Palo Alto, CA: Science and Behavior Books.
Carnap, R. (1950). *Logical foundations of probability*. London, UK: Routledge and Kegan Paul.
Okasha, S. (2016). *Philosophy of science: A very short introduction*. Oxford, UK: Oxford University Press.
Peterfreund, E. (1971). Information, systems, and psychoanalysis. An evolutionary biological approach to psychoanalytic theory. *Psychological Issues* 7 (1), pp.1–397.

Constructing and validating a theoretical model

Chomsky, N. (1957). *Syntactic structures*. The Hague: Mouton.
Chomsky, N. (1965). *Aspects of the theory of syntax*. Cambridge, MA: The MIT Press.
Jaccard, J. and Jacoby, J. (2009). *Theory construction and model-building skills: A practical guide for social scientists*. New York, NY: Guilford.
Richmond, S.A. (1996). A simplification of the theory of simplicity. *Synthese*, 107 (3), pp.373–393.

Human information-processing

Ariel, S. (1987). An information processing theory of family dysfunction. *Psychotherapy, Theory, Research, Practice, Training*, 24 (3S), pp.477–494.
Gibney, P. (2006). The double bind theory: Still crazy-making after all these years. *Psychotherapy in Australia*, 12 (3), pp.48–55.
Lindsay, P.H. and Norman, D.A. (2013). *Human information processing: An introduction to psychology*. New York, NY: Academic Press.
Peterfreund, E. and Schwartz, J.T. (1971) *Information, systems, and psychoanalysis: An evolutionary biological approach to psychoanalytic theory*. New York, NY: International Universities Press.

A unified language of psychotherapy

Ariel, S. (1992). *Strategic family play therapy*. Chichester, UK: Wiley.
Ariel, S. (1999). *Culturally competent family therapy*. Westport, CT: Praeger.
Ariel, S. (2002). *Children's imaginative play: A visit to Wonderland*. Westport, CT: Praeger.

Cybernetics

Cliffe, M.J. (1984). The contribution of cybernetics to the science of psychopathology. *Kybernetes* 13 (2), pp.93–98.

Maltz, M. (2015). *Psycho-cybernetics*. New York, NY: TarcherPerigee.

Semiotics

Ariel, S. (2002). *Children's imaginative play: A visit to Wonderland*. Westport, CT: Praeger.

Cobley, P. and Jansz, L. (2014). *Introducing semiotics: A graphic guide*. London, UK: Icon Books.

The concept of simplicity in the philosophy and methodology of science

Forster, M. (2001). The new science of simplicity. In: Zellner, A., Keuzenkamp, H., and McAleer, M., eds. *Simplicity, inference and modelling*. Cambridge, UK: Cambridge University Press, pp.83–117.

Ladyman, J. (2002). *Understanding philosophy of science*. London, UK: Routledge.

Richmond, S.A. (1996). A simplification of the theory of simplicity. *Synthese*, 107 (3), pp.373–393.

Technical eclecticism

Lazarus, A.A. and Beutler, L.G. (1993). On technical eclecticism. *Journal of Counseling and Development* 71 (4), pp.381–385.

Schaefer, Ch.E. and Drewes, A.A. (2013). *The therapeutic powers of play: 20 core agents of change*. 2nd ed. Hoboken, NJ: Wiley.

Learning and development theories

Bandura, A, (1976). *Social learning theory*. Upper Saddle River, NJ: Prentice-Hall.

Chomsky, N. (2006). *Language and mind*. 3rd ed. Cambridge, UK: Cambridge University press.

Johnson, J.M. (2013). *Radical behaviorism for ABA practitioners*. Cornwall-on-Hudson, NY: Sloan Educational Publishing.

Piaget, J. (1971). *Genetic epistemology*. Translated from the French by E. Duckworth. New York, NY: Norton.

Developmental lines and dimensions

Sigelman, C.K. and Rider, E.A. (2014). *Life-span human development*. 8th ed. Boston, MA: Wadsworth Publishing.

Anatomy and physiology

Mckinley, M. and O'Loughlin, V. (2015). *Anatomy and physiology: An integrative approach*. 2nd ed. New York, NY: McGraw-Hill Education.

Cognitive development

Galotti, K.M. (2016). *Cognitive development: Infancy through adolescence.* 2nd ed. Los Angeles, CA: Sage Publications.
Piaget, J. (2001). *The language and thought of the child.* Translated from French by M. Gabain and R. Gabain. London, UK: Routledge.

Language and its development

Akmajian, A. and Demers, R.A. (2010). *Linguistics: An introduction to language and communication.* 6th ed. Cambridge, MA: MIT Press.
Hoff, E, (2013). *Language development.* 5th ed. Belmont, CA: Wodsworth.
Watzlawick, P. and Helmick Beavin, J. (1967). *Pragmatics of human communication: A study of interactional patterns, pathologies and paradoxes.* New York, NY: Norton.

Emotions

Ariel, S. (2002). *Children's imaginative play: A visit to Wonderland.* Westport, CT: Praeger.
Ekman, P. (2012). *Emotions revealed: Understanding faces and feelings.* London, UK: Weidenfeld & Nicolson.
Gross, J.J., ed. (2015). *Handbook of emotion regulation.* 2nd ed. New York, NY: Guilford.
Feldman B.L. (2017). *How emotions are made: The secret life of the brain.* Boston, MA: Houghton Mifflin Harcourt.

Self and body image and concept, gender identity

Bracken, B. (1995). *Handbook of self-concept: Developmental, social and clinical considerations.* Hoboken, NJ: Wiley.
Cullari, S., Vosburgh, M., Shotwell, A., Inzodda, J. and Davenport, W. (2002). Body-image assessment: A review and evaluation of a new computer-aided measurement technique. *North American Journal of Psychology* 4 (2), pp.221–232.
Owen Blackmore, J.E. and Berenbaum, Sh.A. (2008). *Gender development.* Hove, UK: Psychology Press.

Object relations, ego and self-development

Blanck, G. and Blanck, R. (1974). *Ego psychology: Theory and practice.* New York, NY: Columbia University Press.
Greenspan, S.I. (1989). *Development of the ego: Implications for personality theory, psychopathology and the psychotherapeutic process.* Madison, CT: International Universities Press.
Klein, M. (1935). *The psychoanalysis of children.* London, UK: Hogarth Press.
Kohut, H. (1971). *The analysis of the self.* New York, NY: International Universities Press.
Kohut, H. and Wolf, E.S. (1978). The disorders of the self and their treatment: An outline. *The International Journal of Psychoanalysis* 59, pp.413–425.
Lessem, P.A. (2012). *Self psychology: An introduction.* New York, NY: Jason Aronson.

Scharff, D.E. (1995). *Object relations theory and practice: An introduction*. New York, NY: Jason Aronson.

St.Clair, M. and Wigren, J. (2003). *Object relations and self-psychology: An introduction*. 4th ed. Boston, MA: Brooks Cole.

Body and self-boundaries

Mahler, M.S., Fine, F. and Bergman, A. (2008). *The psychological birth of the human infant: Symbiosis and individuation*. Reprint. New York, NY: Basic Books.

Attachment

Wallin, D.J. (2015). *Attachment in psychotherapy*. New York, NY: Guilford.

Empathy

Coplan, A. and Goldie, P., eds. (2011). *Empathy: Philosophical and psychological perspectives*. Oxford, UK: Oxford University Press.

Psychosexual development

Moll, A. (2016). *The sexual life of the child: A study into psychosexual development and the stages of puberty*. Charleston, SC: CreateSpace Independent Publishing Platform.

Moral development

Killen, M and Smetana, J.G., eds. *Handbook of moral development*. 2nd ed. Hove, UK: Psychology Press.

Part 2

X-raying make-believe play

Chapter 4

Play observation techniques

Make-believe play is a semiotic system, a language in the wide sense of the term. Like every language, the language of make-believe play has universal features, applying to every manifestation of make-believe play everywhere, and local features, found in the make-believe play of specific individuals or groups, in specific times and places. Every play therapist is advised to learn the language of make-believe play, its universal and local features, in order to be able to understand the make-believe play of the clients, decipher its manifest and hidden meanings and communicative functions, and communicate with the clients in their own play language. The following chapters include concepts and tools for describing and analyzing observed make-believe play as a semiotic system.

Observations on spontaneous play and non-play behavior

Observations of the play or non-play behavior of an individual adult or child, a family or a group are conducted before the therapy as a part of the pre-therapy diagnostic evaluation and, continuously, during all therapy sessions.

When possible, an observation can be videotaped, and if impossible, it can be recorded by hand. Observations and recording techniques are introduced in detail in Ariel (1992, 1999, 2002 and 2018). Below only some of the main features of these techniques are presented.

What we record in our observation protocol is the *raw material* of the observed behavior, that is, what can be directly grasped by our senses. The raw material includes the following expressive media: *vocal–linguistic* (speech and various other sounds produced by the observed players), *spatial* (the use of space by the observed players), *motional* (the gestures and facial expressions produced by the players) and *tactile* (touching oneself, other players or objects).

Characteristic errors in recording observations are interpretation and generalizations instead of a detailed objective description of the raw materials and ignoring non-verbal behavior.

Interdisciplinary seminar

Ethan: I have to get used to observing and transcribing play and non-play behavior in such minute detail. So far, in my practice, I have used mainly my intuition. I did generalize and mix observation with interpretation. I still have to be convinced that a microscopic observation is preferable to global observation.

Shlomo: When we watch a child play, we see and hear a very small portion of the observed behavior, and tend to invent, unconsciously, things that did not occur at all. We are also likely to miss details that are crucial to understanding what was going on in the play. All the more so if it is a family or a group play.

Let's do an experiment. I put on the table a random collection of toys, dolls and other objects I brought with me. Lailah and Ethan, you will play freely with these objects and I will videotape your play. Daniel and Anna, you will watch their play and record what you see and hear in as much detail as possible. Then we'll watch the video and compare what you've recorded with what we see on the video.

(Lailah and Ethan start playing. After three minutes Shlomo tells them to stop.)

Shlomo: OK, Daniel, what did you write?
Daniel: Ethan made a toy kick a ball.
Shlomo: What kind of toy?
Daniel: I think a doll of a guy in a soccer player's uniform.
Shlomo: Which way did he kick the ball?
Daniel: I think in the general direction of Lailah. I'm not sure. There was a toy table there. I think he played as if it was the soccer gate. Then Lailah made a man's doll sit on a chair, led two dolls on the table and said something in Arabic.
Shlomo: Can you describe the doll she seated on a chair?
Daniel: I think it was an old man.
Shlomo: And the two dolls?
Daniel: I'm not sure.
Shlomo: What did she make the two dolls do?
Daniel: Walk. Then they stopped walking.
Shlomo: OK, let's watch the video. Daniel, I'll run the video and stop every few seconds. You'll say out loud what you see and hear. After each short while I'll stop the video, so you can see, hear and talk.
Daniel: Lailah holds a doll of a bearded man in her left hand and tries to seat it on a toy chair. Now I see why I thought it was an old man. The doll has a beard, but it is black, doesn't seem to be a doll of an old man. Ethan holds a young man's doll in his right hand and a small rubber ball in his left hand. Now I see that the guy's doll doesn't wear a soccer uniform but long trousers and a hat. He rolls the ball toward the foot of the guy's doll and the guy kicks the ball towards Lailah's man with the beard, not toward the table, which is placed on the right side. Lailah doesn't pay attention to the ball. She takes a

woman's doll in her hand and a man's doll in her left hand and places them in front of the man with the beard. Now |I see it was a man and a woman. She didn't make them walk, just to stand facing the man with the beard. She says something in Arabic in a woman's voice and then something in Arabic in what is supposed to be a man's voice. Ethan takes the ball and makes the guy kick the ball toward Lailah's toys more forcefully. Lailah still ignores the ball. She takes a plastic toy ear and holds it to the left ear of the man with the beard. I see I missed the ear thing. Ethan makes the guy's doll turn his back on Lailah's toys.

Shlomo: OK, that will do.

Ethan: I can see your point now, Shlomo. Daniel saw only a part of what had happened in the play and projected on the play things that fit his mind set, like saw a football game and imagined a kick in the direction of the table and all that.

Shlomo: Ethan and Lailah, can you tell us what you did in your play and what you were thinking and feeling while doing it?

Lailah: I saw the bearded man doll. In my imagination he was a Qadi, a Muslim judge. I made him sit on a chair which I imagined was a judge's bench. Then a husband and wife stood before him to consult with him about the possibility of reaching reconciliation or getting divorce. I know where I took this scene from. My sister and her husband do not get along and she wants to get divorced. It's very hard for me to accept it. I am really worried about her. Then I made the woman speak Arabic in a weak, small voice because of the shame. The Qadi could barely hear her, so I put a toy ear on his ear to signal an effort to hear. I think at this point I was influenced by something else. My father has recently had a hearing loss and he needs a hearing aid. That worries me too. He's too young to lose hearing.

Anna: Yes, it's sad, it's really sad when things are not what they used to be. It's amazing how we project out emotional concerns on the play. But I would have never guessed the meaning of the play for you, Lailah. How can one understand the meaning of the play if the player doesn't explain his content as you did?

Shlomo: Yes, interpreting play or behavior in general is not simple at all. We will discuss this in our next sessions.

Ethan: You've completely forgotten about me. (He makes a sad face.) I wanted Lailah, or her dolls, to play soccer with me. I felt lonely and needed company. I know soccer is men's game.

Shlomo: Not in the USA.

Lailah: I was so preoccupied with my play that I didn't notice the ball at all.

Ethan: I tried harder, but when you again didn't respond, I felt frustrated and angry and turned my back on you, hoping that you would notice and react at last. All this is half-joking of course.

Shlomo: This experience shows how play can be an excellent tool in family or group therapy. We will discuss this in our next sessions.

Summary of chapter 4

Make-believe play is a language, a semiotic system. Observations of spontaneous make-believe play in various stages of the play therapy are a rich source of diagnostic information. A play therapist who possesses tools for observing and interpreting the clients' play can better understand the case and communicate with the players in their own play language. The observer must focus on and record the play at the raw material level, while trying to absorb as many verbal–vocal, spatial, motional and tactile details as possible. This is not at all an easy task. Interpretations and generalization should be postponed to a later stage. The formulation of the protocol in a natural language cannot be accurate.

Assignments

1. Perform a series of verbal and non-verbal play acts. Describe, speaking aloud, your own verbal and non-verbal actions in great detail, while performing them. In your verbal descriptions refer to all the vocal and sound, spatial, motional, facial expressions and touch aspects of your actions, like in this example, "I am inserting my right hand into a glove puppet of a monkey, using my left hand to get the puppet on my right hand. I am raising my left arm with the palm facing downwards, above my head. I am raising my right arm with a fast and abrupt movement and am placing the monkey puppet on the palm of my left hand. I am making the monkey puppet jump up and down above the palm of my left hand three time and while making it jump fast, I am making a choking voice, by inhaling fast, and then am saying, in the same way, by inhaling, 'I am Cheetah!'"

    If you are with other people, do the same exercise with one person doing the action and another person doing the verbal description simultaneously.

    Observe two children play with toys. Write a detailed description of their activity for five minutes.
2. This exercise can also be done with adults (e.g. peer trainees) playing with toys.
3. Videotape short samples of spontaneous play activities of two children. Prepare transcription sheets and write the videotaped activities into the sheets.

A classified list of publications

Observation and recording techniques

Ariel, S. (1992). *Strategic family play therapy*. Chichester, UK: Wiley.
Ariel, S. (1999). *Culturally competent family therapy*. Westport, CT: Praeger.

Ariel, S. (2002). *Children's imaginative play: A visit to Wonderland*. Westport, CT: Praeger.
Ariel, S. (2018). *Multi-dimensional therapy with families, children and adults*. London, UK: Routledge.
Benzten, W.R. (2008). *Seeing young children: A guide to observing and recording behavior*. Belmont, CA: Wadsworth Cengage Learning.
Cohen, D. H., Stern, V., Balaban, N. and Gropper, N. (2015). *Observing and recording the behavior of young children*. 6th Edition. New York, NY: Teachers College Press.

Chapter 5

Microscopic analysis of observed play

Once the observed play has been recorded on the raw-material level, it can be interpreted and analyzed on the semantic and pragmatic levels. In the first stage, the interpretation and analysis are microscopic, involving the identification and interpretation of the minimal units out of which the play is composed, its building blocks. In the second stage, the analysis is macroscopic, which includes a description of the structural and functional relations between the different units at the three levels, in other words, the patterns, the rules underlying the details. The observed make-believe play can be viewed as a text, which we are trying to understand and discover the deep structures lying behind its surface.

Interdisciplinary seminar

Microscopic analysis

Shlomo: Play behavior on the raw material level includes the following media: vocal–linguistic, spatial, motional and tactile. On the semantic level, private thoughts and feelings that are signified by these media are described. The uses of semantically interpreted raw material entities in actual verbal and non-verbal contexts are described on the pragmatic level. Of particular importance for our purposes are pragmatic uses in interpersonal communication, both between the players and between characters in the play that are represented, for instance, by puppets. Consider for instance the following play episode:

Observation 5.1 Ava and Grace
In kindergarten, Ava (5.6) puts dolls representing all sorts of animals in a corner of the room and surrounds the corner with toy chairs. She "feeds" the animals with colored plastic balls. Grace (5.3) makes a woman doll and a girl doll approach the surrounding area and says, as if from the mouth of the

woman doll, "I brought my daughter to the zoo. may I come in?" Ava says, "No, the zoo is closed to visitors. Now we feed the animals."

Let's analyze this play on the three levels of analysis.

Ethan: On the raw material level we have Grace saying, "I brought my daughter, etc." in an adult woman's voice. Ava is saying, "No, the zoo is closed, etc.", apparently in a resolute adult voice. That's vocal–linguistic. Spatial – Ava created her own territory by circling "the zoo" with little chairs and didn't let Grace and her dolls enter this territory. Motional – Ava put little plastic dolls near the animals' mouths, probably also tactile. Grace moved the woman and girl dolls toward "the zoo". Is it also tactile, because she touches her dolls?

Shlomo: No, because she has to hold the dolls in order to move them. Touching them is not a part of the make-believe play. It's just a technical necessity.

Anna: The semantic level? Something like "This is my zoo, not yours."

Shlomo: This statement belongs to the pragmatic level, not to the semantic level, because it is an instant of interpersonal communication. Anyway, at this stage we don't go to such a level of generalization.

Lailah: On the semantic level, in Ava's play, I would say something like nurturing?

Shlomo: Again, Lailah, this is an over-generalization. I mean much simpler things, like, "The space surrounded by toy chairs on the raw material level signifies a zoo on the semantic level"; "Surrounding the zoo by little chairs on the raw material level signifies the zoo's fence on the semantic level"; "A toy lion on the raw material level signifies a lion on the semantic level"; "Putting a small plastic ball near the mouth of a toy giraffe on the raw material level signifies feeding the giraffe on the semantic level", etc.

Daniel: On the pragmatic level, the zoo's fence conveys an interpersonal communication message such as, "This is my territory and you are not allowed to get in without my permission" Is that right?

Shlomo: Yes. This is a message from Ava to Grace. But on the pragmatic level one can also describe communication between the imaginary characters in the play, e.g. "Visitors cannot be admitted to the zoo at this time."

We should distinguish between a microscopic analysis and a macroscopic analysis.

Microscopic analysis breaks the behavior into minimal units at each level. Macroscopic analysis looks for relations between such units, syntactic relations, recurring patterns, regularities, rules.

Anna: It seems that semantically interpreted units are like words in a language or something like that.

Shlomo: Yes, or meaningful parts of words. Now, on the pragmatic level, the units are not minimal semantically interpreted units but sequencing of such units that convey a single message, like sentences in a language. I call such sequences *structures*.

Ethan: Let me try. In Grace's play, the sequence "She makes a woman doll and a girl doll approach the surrounded area and says, as if from the mouth of the woman doll, 'I brought my daughter to the zoo. May I come in?'" Is this a structure? It includes both motional and spatial raw materials and verbal–linguistic raw materials, but more than one sentence.

Shlomo: The comparison to sentences is not one-to-one. Does it convey a single communicative message?

Ethan: Yes, finding out whether she and her daughter can be admitted to the zoo.

Shlomo: Yes. I would like to introduce two terms that can help us analyze communicative messages on the pragmatic level: *Presupposition* and *purpose*. For example, Ava presupposed that Grace's purpose was to invade her territory. Ava's purpose was to prevent her from achieving her purpose. What were Grace's presupposition and purpose?

Anna: Her presupposition was that if she asks for permission, then Ava will let her in.

Shlomo: This is not a presupposition, it is a prediction.

Anna: I'm not sure I see the difference.

Shlomo: Presupposition is not about predicting your addressee's response if you act in a certain way. It is about what you assume about the addressee's current state of mind or purpose.

Daniel: Maybe Grace's presupposition was that Ava had not made up her mind whether she wanted her in her territory or not. On the basis of this presupposition she decided which message to convey and hoped (or predicted) that Ava would consent.

Shlomo: Yes. The transmitter of a message acts upon his or her presupposition with a view to achieving his or her purpose, which usually has to do with *proximity* and *control*. Grace's purpose was proximity and Ava's purpose was distance and control.

I'd like to add that presuppositions are often wrong, or, to use a term we learned in a previous session, bugged, and therefore the purpose is likely to be bugged too.

Ethan: These terms begin to invade my dreams.

Shlomo: There will be more.

Summary of chapter 5

The first stage of the interpretation and analysis of observed and recorded make-believe play is microscopic analysis, identifying the building blocks of the observed play on the raw material, semantic and pragmatic levels. Minimal units on the raw material and semantic levels level are combinations of vocal–linguistic, spatial, motional and tactile features that carry meaning on the semantic level. It is minimal if it cannot be broken down to smaller units without losing its meaning. Minimal units on the pragmatic level are structures, that is, sequences of semantically interpreted raw material units that have a single communicative message.

Key concepts in analyzing structures are purpose (the kind of interpersonal message the player wants to convey by his or her play structure) and presupposition (the way the player understands the message conveyed by the play structure produced by his or her play partner). The purpose is influenced by the presupposition.

Assignments

Do a microscopic analysis of the following observation, using the concepts and techniques introduced in this chapter.

Observation 5.2 Shay and Gal
Shay (7) and Gal (6.10) play in Shay's room. Shay is sitting on the floor wearing a motorcycle helmet. He takes off the helmet and puts on a clown hat. Then he picks up a toy rabbit and makes it walk toward Gal, who is holding a toy horse.

Shay: I can jump higher than the horse (making the rabbit leap over the horse). You know why? Because I have long ears and I eat carrot.
Gal: And I eat grass.
Shay: I can run faster than you. Let's do a running race.
    Gal is making his horse run. Shay doesn't join him.
Gal: You can't run at all, you can only jump. And now I'm going to kick you and I won't be your friend.
    Shay is putting on the helmet.
Shay: You can't kick me.
Gal: I can.
    Shay is taking off the helmet and is putting on the clown hat.
Shay: I am a clown in a circus. I'm trying to run and then I keep falling.

Shay is running and falling.
    Gal is picking up a toy elephant. He is saying, "The elephant will splash water from his trunk and will make a puddle. And then the horse will try to leap over the puddle and will fall into the water."
    Shay and Gal are laughing.

A classified list of publications

Semantics and pragmatics

Ariel, S. (1992). *Strategic family play therapy*. Chichester, UK: Wiley.
Ariel, S. (1997). *Culturally competent family therapy*. Westport, CT: Praeger.

Ariel, S. (2002). *Children's imaginative play: A visit to Wonderland.* Westport, CT: Praeger.
Ariel, S. (2018). *Multi-dimensional therapy with families, children and adults: The Diamond Model.* London, UK: Routledge.
Chandler, D. (2017). *Semiotics: The basics.* London, UK: Routledge.
Hornsby, D. (2014). *Linguistics – a complete introduction: A teach yourself guide.* New York, NY: McGraw-Hill Education.
Huang, Y. (2015). *Pragmatics.* Oxford, UK: Oxford University Press.
Kearns, K. (2011). *Semantics.* London, UK: Palgrave.

Chapter 6
Macroscopic analysis on the semantic level

As stated in Chapter 5, a microscopic analysis of an observation involves parsing the raw material play sequences into minimal meaningful units, that is, units that carry thematic and emotive meanings on the semantic level. Microscopic analysis on the pragmatic level consists of identifying chains of semantically interpreted raw material units (*structures*) that convey an interpersonal message. A macroscopic analysis on the semantic level searches for syntactic relations between semantically interpreted units. It looks for regularities and recurring patterns, like the rules of a language.

Context Dependent Componential Analysis

Componential Analysis is a technique developed by anthropological linguists as a method for revealing and describing semantic systems, i.e. covert inter-relations among meaning dimensions of words in various "exotic" languages. (Hammel, 1965). Context Dependent Componential Analysis (CDCA) is my own elaboration of this technique. It can be applied to any sample of observed behavior, especially individual or interpersonal play behavior, or to any text such as a verbal interview. The need to contextualize the original technique was motivated by the necessity to perform macroscopic analyses of unconventional behaviors. In analyzing the underlying dimensions of such behaviors, we rely less on the conventional knowledge we have about language and culture, and more on attempting to learn the private verbal and non-verbal behavior of the people we observe. A child engaged in make-believe play does not necessarily use raw material and semantic units in the ways they are commonly used in her culture or society. She can introduce in her play a dragon toy, but from the contexts in which she uses this toy one can learn that she created in her private world something different from a conventional dragon. The dragon in her play is much more a frightened little baby than a monster. Such private raw material signs and signified meanings can be understood only if the contexts in which they occur are taken into account, hence the need for CDCA. With the aid of CDCA, the contextualized uses of both raw material units and semantic units are systematically categorized into sets, defined by dimensions and sub-dimensions. The final result of each such analysis is a map exhibiting the hierarchical patterns of relations between the various signifying (raw-material) dimensions and signified (semantic) dimensions and sub-dimensions. These hierarchical patterns are cross-classified with the degrees of emotional intensities associated with the various dimensions and sub-dimensions. Such a map constitutes a partial description of the deep, covert structures underlying the observed play behavior or a text. It is a kind of x-ray picture of the emotion-balancing mechanisms that underlie the observed play behavior, and a kind of dictionary of the observed person's private play language. CDCA helps us communicate with the clients in their own private play language. Furthermore, it facilitates the further discovery and formulation of more rules representing hidden patterns lying behind the surface of the observed verbal and non-verbal play behavior.

A full demonstration of the CDCA technique is beyond the scope of this book. Such a full demonstration is found in Ariel (2002, 2018). To give an idea of what some of the CDCA discovery procedures and the final map look like, let me show how CDCA could be applied to the following observation. The following illustration applies just to the semantic level, although CDCA can be performed on the raw material level too.

Observation 6.1 Tamar
Five-year-old Tamar is painting a girl's image with watercolors on a sheet of paper, which is placed on a newspaper. The sheet is too small to include the whole figure, so she paints the head and feet on the newspaper. She is saying,

"They painted me with watercolors and then I became huge and beautiful."

She looks at me coquettishly, flinging her arms forward and moving her body gracefully, as if displaying her beauty.

She takes a dragon doll lying beside her on the table and says, "Now they turned me into a huge dragon and I was really scaring people. And I had huge nails and it was very scary."

She turns the dragon doll toward dolls placed on the table, moves the dragon with sharp attacking gestures, exposing her teeth and making a throaty growl.

She is saying, "It was just a disguise. I was very happy, because they didn't know it was me. But they locked me in a high tower and my mother came to rescue me and then when we went home, they knew it was me and then they understood."

She is getting off the chair and goes under the table. She is saying, "And then we lived happily at home, but they were looking for me because daddy was not home, and he was worried."

She comes out from under the table and hides under a big pillow. She is saying, "And then I got lost and it was great fun."

She rolls on the floor and lies still, saying, "But once an old woman killed me and then they killed her too."

She gets up and walks around the room. She is saying, "And then I liked to go places all the time and my daddy and mommy came to where I was getting lost and then I was very worried."

She sits down on the pillow that previously she lay beneath. She is saying, "And then daddy and mommy came to where I was, and they found me there and then I went home with them and I loved myself."

I will not present here the steps of the CDCA of this observation, just the final results of its full analysis.

I use the term *emotive* to denote a central emotional concern, in other words, a theme strongly associated in a person's mind with specific emotions. The concept of emotive will be discussed in detail further below and in Chapter 11.

The main emotive underlying Tamar's play, as shown by the CDCA, was, *fear of one's own fantasies of power and independence*. The results of the CDCA are displayed in Table 6.1.

This table holds a great deal of information. It presents what seems to be one of Tamar's central emotional concerns (emotives), and the mechanism of emotion-balancing applying to this emotive and its sub-dimensions, or sub-emotives. The central emotive seems to be her own fantasies of power and independence. The sub-dimensions (sub-emotives) represent different aspects of these fantasies and the associated fears: power over others, aggression, and independence or autonomy. Typically for Tamar's age and level of development, she examines, mainly in fantasy, the limits of her own power. The basic conflict is between her aspiration to be big and strong ("huge"), win in an imaginary beauty contest, show her power, deal on her own with aggression and violence directed against her, establish her own self-identity and be independent and autonomous, less attached to her parents. However, being only five years old, she is sharply aware of her own powerlessness and dependence. These fantasies frighten her. When the fear increases, she brings to her play contents in which she is not conceived as so powerful and

Table 6.1 Semantic CDCA of Observation 6.1 (Tamar)

The intensity of fear	High	Medium	Low
Subdimensions			
Power over others vs. Powerlessness	punished (locked up);	ugly (dragon); normal size (girl);	showing off beauty; huge size (girl, dragon); scaring (dragon);
Aggression vs. Tameness	killed (by old woman);	saved, protected (by parents, at home); disguised;	killing (old woman); attacking (dragon); real identity;
Independence vs. Dependence	getting lost involuntarily;	parents worried parents looking for;	getting lost by free will; hiding (fun);
Free will and Attachment		parents found;	wandering (by choice); happy at home;

independent but needs parental figures to save and protect her. "They" in her play represent internal figures within her own psyche, which both empower her (paint her as huge and beautiful, turn her into a huge, scary dragon) but also punish her for being too powerful, subdue and tame her by locking her, like the rebellious princess in fairy tales, in a high tower. "They" accept her when they see her real, undisguised, non-threatening identity. "They" kill the old woman (a fairy tale witch) who "killed her" and help her parents find her when she gets lost.

Tamar's play on the semantic level may be seen as a series of fluctuations between the high fear, medium fear and no fear, related to the various sub-dimensions of her central emotive: fear of her own fantasies of power. The fluctuations are defenses against the fear. When the fear associated with a specific type of theme increases, she moves on to a less frightening theme, calms down, gathers strength and returns to the previous type of theme. This is a cybernetic emotion-balancing mechanism that will be discussed in detail in Chapter 11. When she shows off her beauty and her big size, she is punished by being turned into an ugly but still huge dragon, and when the dragon acts aggressively and scares people, it is being subdued and locked up. But then "they" realized that she wasn't really a dragon, just a nice girl in disguise, so they understood and took a positive stance. When she is in trouble, locked up, her mother saves her. When she is "killed" by the old woman, "they" kill the old woman. She fluctuates between voluntarily getting lost, hiding and taking solitary walks on the one hand and realizing that her parents worry about her, that she can really get lost. So, her parents find her and take her back home where she is sheltered, protected and loved.

Table 6.1 can also serve as a kind of dictionary, defining the main private signified contents in Tamar's make-believe play and their emotional valence. For example, it can be seen from examining this table that "getting lost" has a double meaning in Tamar's play: Independence, associated with a low level of fear of "being" powerful, on the one hand; and dependence, associated with a high level of fear of "being" powerful, on the other hand. "Dragon" means aggression associated with a low level of fear of being powerful, and so forth.

Interdisciplinary seminar

Shlomo: CDCA is not a mechanical procedure but a heuristic procedure, that is, a procedure serving as an aid to analyzing data and solve problems. A table like Table 6.1 is an idiographic theory about the underlying structure of the play's semantic contents. An idiographic theory is a theory about a specific case.

Lailah: Can one create a valid idiographic theory that is based just on a three minute observation?

Shlomo: I applied CDCA to a brief observation just to demonstrate the technique. In reality, the technique will be applied to a larger play sample or to several samples, although even applying it to a very brief observation yield a considerable amount of information.

Ethan: But the procedure is time-consuming and tedious. Are we expected to do a CDCA in each case we are supposed to treat?

Shlomo: No, but one can construct such a chart without going through all the stages of the analysis, just by examining the observation carefully, using logic, creativity and intuition. To test the validity of the results of our CDCA, we can compare alternative results of a CDCA of the same data sample, and prefer the simpler one, that is the more comprehensive, parsimonious, consistent and plausible one. We can also examine more samples of the play of the same player and see whether our preferred CDCA applies to them – predictive validity.

Daniel: But in other samples the player will produce different contents, won't they?

Shlomo: The CDCA will not predict the same contents but the same or similar thematic structure of the contents, whatever they are. Let us look at another sample of Tamar's play and see whether the results of our CDCA apply to it.

Observation 6.2 Tamar

Tamar places on the table a puppet of a pink unicorn with golden horns and by its side a brown monkey doll. She addresses me, saying, "This is Unicorney and this is Monkey-Monkey." She puts on the table a doll of a yellow teddy-bear and tells me, "This is the silly bear."

She wears pink fairy wings and is holding a pink fairy magic wand.

She says, "Unicorney and Monkey-Monkey come to the princess and ask her who is more beautiful."

I'm asking her, "Where is the princess?"

She says, "I'm half a fairy and half a princess."

She asks, as if from the mouths of the unicorn and the monkey, "Princess-fairy, who of the two of us is more beautiful?"

She strokes the hair of the unicorn and is saying in a soft voice, "You are beautiful, Unicorney."

Then she looks at the monkey doll without touching it and says, "And you are ugly." She adds, "But Monkey-Monkey is not really Monkey-Monkey. He just disguised himself as Monkey-Monkey. What he really is, is Bamboli. Bamboli is beautiful."

She takes a girl's doll and seats her on the teddy-bear's knees.

She says in "a bear's voice", "Little princess, why do you put on socks and only then shoes. You should first put on shoes and only then socks."

She is rubbing the neck of the girl's doll with the magic wand, saying, "The silly bear is telling her that she should be thrown into the pool and drown, but he thinks the floor is a pool."

She inserts a baby doll under her shirt and says, "Now she is being born and it doesn't hurt. O no! The silly bear told the baby princess to eat soap and now she is sick and should stay in the hospital for three days."

She picks an old woman doll and says, "This is the nurse in the hospital."

She lays the baby doll on the table and covers her with a piece of cloth. Then she picks up the baby doll, inserts her under her shirt, puts the girl's doll mouth close to her nipple and says, "Now she is sucking milk and she will be well again."

She walks to the other side of the room, takes a shoe box and lays the baby doll inside it. She is walking slowly toward me, talking to me in a very sad voice, "I want to tell you something very sad. Our baby is dead. I forgot her in the middle of the street and a car ran over her. But you are not angry, are you?"

She brings the old woman doll ("nurse") close to the baby doll in the box. The old woman bows her head at the baby doll and says, "She is breathing! Quickly! Breast-feed her and she'll be fine!"

Daniel: Many of the themes of Observation 6.1 also appear in Observation 6.2 – beauty, aggression, death. Other themes found in Observation 6.1 don't exist in Observation 6.2, such as getting lost and found, being locked up, etc.

Shlomo: Observation 6.2 was conducted a month after Observation 6.1. You are right. In a CDCA of Observation 6.2 the sub-dimension of independence vs. dependence and attachment would not be included. But what about the central emotive and the other sub-dimensions?

Ethan: It seems that in Observation 6.2 the central emotive is again fear of her own fantasies of power. In a CDCA of Observation 6.2 the sub-dimensions of power over others and aggression would be included too. The fairy-princess has the authority to serve as a judge in a beauty contest. She rejects the ugly Monkey-Monkey. But then she can't deal emotionally with her own power and invents the idea that the monkey's ugliness was just a disguise.

Anna: Like the dragon in Observation 6.1, who was just disguised as a dragon. I discern guilt here. She also blames herself for the baby's death.

Daniel: She is afraid of the responsibility for other's well-being, happiness, health and even life.

Shlomo: Let us try to apply CDCA to the following observation. Again, we will not go through the formal stages of the analysis. Just use your creativity and intuition and put the final results in a tabular form, like Table 6.1.

Observation 6.3 Jonathan
Jonathan (7.6) places a big toy dinosaur on the table. He takes the bee toys, moves them in the air and hums.

He says, "Dinosaurs hate bees because they don't like their stings."

He makes the bees fly away from the dinosaur, saying, "The bees run away, because bees are afraid of dinosaurs, because they can devour them."

He picks up a crocodile toy, saying, "The crocodile is not afraid of the bees as much as the dinosaur is afraid of them because his skin is hard."

He flings the bees at the crocodile and says in a humming voice, "Your skin won't protect you. If you swallow us, we'll sting you inside your body! We've already stung a lot of dinosaurs, even a real dragon, even though we don't like fire. But we are not afraid of fire or smoke, even though it hurts the eyes, but our eyes are hard and the smoke can't penetrate them, and we can fly high. We can fly even with our eyes closed. Besides, our sting is poisonous but it is not poisonous for dinosaurs, but it hurts."

He makes the crocodile whisper to the dinosaur, "Let's make them a nectar trap."

He makes the bees fly closer to the crocodile and dinosaur. They say in a humming voice, "We heard you! We heard You! You won't catch us!"

Anna: Is the central emotive *fear of one's own fantasies of power?* Seems like it is. Are the main sub-dimensions *power over others* and *aggression*? Seems like they are. But I don't think the subdimension independence is relevant in this observation.

Ethan: Where do you see fear of one's own power in Jonathan's play? He doesn't seem to have any fear-arousing emotional conflict around power. He enjoys the power struggles.

Shlomo: Anna, you have asked yourself whether the emotives and sub-emotives we found in Tamar's play also apply to Jonathan's play. Forget about the CDCA of Tamar's play. It is irrelevant to Jonathan's play. We apply CDCA case-by-case. The results of the CDCA of the play of one player can be radically different from those of another player.

Anna: OK. Now I understand.

Shlomo: Take your time. Try to create a table representing the results of the CDCA of Jonathan's play, using logic, creativity and intuition.

(The four are working, consulting one another from time to time.)

Lailah: We got to something. Hope we were on the right track. The central emotive manifested in Jonathan's play is "fear of being physically hurt by an enemy".

(They present Table 6.2, shown on the next page.)

Shlomo: Excellent! Good work.

Anna: I don't know why we talk about fear. Jonathan seemed to enjoy playing the battle between the bees and the other animals, he wasn't afraid at all.

Shlomo: That's the beauty of play. Since the world of play is not a real world, players can materialize in their make-believe play things that frighten them in real life.

Daniel: And excite them too. Not only in play people overcome fear by engaging in scary, challenging activities, e.g. extreme sports.

Shlomo: But play cannot always make it possible to overcome fears. When a child expresses very difficult contents in his or her play, for example post-traumatic contents, the play can stop being fun. It can arouse intense fears, even re-traumatize the player. In such cases, we must help the child use the play as an instrument for achieving emotional balance. We will return to this subject in our next sessions.

Lailah: What other therapeutic goals does our semantic analysis serve?

Shlomo: It helps us communicate with the player in his or her own play language. For example, if we understand the role of disguise in Tamar's play as a means of overcoming her fear of excessive use of her own power, we can use disguise as a theme in play therapy with Tamar.

Table 6.2 Semantic CDCA of Observation 6.3 (Jonathan)

The intensity of fear	High	Medium	Low
Subdimensions			
Degree of injury	poisonous stinging;	poisonous stinging (of dinosaur, only hurts); hurt by dragon's fire; devouring (by dinosaur); can be stung inside;	eyes hurt by smoke; devouring (by crocodile);
Vulnerability vs. immunity	inside body;	flying away; closing eyes (against smoke);	impenetrable (skin of crocodile, eyes of bees);
Tactical collaboration	bees near plot;		nectar trap, bees collaborate;

Summary of chapter 6

A macroscopic analysis searches for syntactic relations between minimal raw material, semantic and pragmatic units and structures that have been identified by a microscopic analysis. It looks for regularities and recurring patterns, like the rules of a language. A heuristic semantic macroscopic analysis, Context Dependent Componential Analysis (CDCA), is presented and illustrated. This technique is a modified version of Componential Analysis, developed by anthropological linguists for studying semantic systems in various cultures. It is contextualized because children in their make-believe play often assign raw material units unconventional meanings, that can be understood only by examining the contexts in which these units are used. CDCA leads toward displaying the basic semantic components underlying a make-believe play text, cross-classified with respect to emotive-related emotional intensity. CDCA exposes the play's emotive-related emotion-balancing mechanism and also serves as a kind of "dictionary", defining the private meanings of the player's semantic contents.

Assignments

1. Why is CDCA context-dependent?
2. What are the benefits of CDCA for a play therapist?
3. Do a CDCA of Rusella's play in Session 1.1 (Rusella).

A classified list of publications

Creating and validating an idiographic theory

Ariel, S. (2018). *Multi-dimensional therapy with families, children and adults: The Diamond Model*. London, UK: Routledge.

Chomsky, N. (2015). *Syntactic structures*. Eastford, CT: Marino Fine Books.

Semiotics

Cobley, P. and Jansz, L. (2014). *Introducing semiotics: A graphic guide*. London, UK: Icon Books.

Semantics

Saeed, J.I. (2015). *Semantics,* Fourth edition. Hoboken, NJ: Wiley-Blackwell.

Componential analysis

Ariel, S. (2002). *Children's imaginative play: A visit to Wonderland*. Westport, CT: Praeger.

Hammel, E.A., ed. (1965). Formal semantic analysis. Special publication, *American Anthropologist*, 67(5).

Chapter 7
Macroscopic analysis on the pragmatic level

Inter-relations between individuals and groups of humans and animals revolve around proximity and control. Such inter-relations have manifold manifestations.

One of the functions of make-believe play is to shift negotiations and conflicts around proximity or control to the world of imagination, thereby reducing the danger that the conflict could deteriorate into physical or verbal violence or into a rupture between the parties. The players have a tacit mutual agreement to transfer their proximity-control conflicts to the realm of make-believe. The playful negotiation tactics employed by children are unique to make-believe play and belong to its very special bag of tricks. Since in make-believe play children are at least partly free of the chains of reality and social conventions, they are at liberty to draw uncommonly rich, flexible and sophisticated devices from this bag. The following observation includes a whole range of such devices.

Observation 7.1 Easy riders
Two five-year-old girls, Dana and Ruttie, play in their kindergarten playground. Dana approaches a blue metal tube mounted on stands, which serves as a kind of crawling tunnel. She calls, "Ruttie! Let's go up on this horse!" She mounts the tube and sits on it astride, moving her legs alternately, slowly, forward and backward, "riding".

Ruttie ignores Dana's invitation to ride together. After a short while, Dana calls "Halt!" and stops moving her legs. She looks at Ruttie and makes an inviting gesture with an arm. Ruttie mounts on the "horse", but instead of sitting behind Dana, as might be expected, she is sitting astride in front of her, calling out, "Go!" and begins moving her legs swiftly, as if galloping. Then she is calling, "Let's pretend the baby is in front and the mommy is behind. Let's pretend the mommy allowed her baby to get lost, because she had a dog. When babies get lost, the dog brings them back. Come on! You got home and told your baby, 'Cutie, you are allowed to get lost'. Are you gonna get off the horse then?"

Dana co-operates. She is climbing off the "horse" and is saying, "OK, I'm going home."

Ruttie is calling, "Mommy! Get me this bag. I need it, and the blanket too". Dana cannot find "a bag" and "a blanket", so Ruttie is climbing off the "horse". She is going to a junk case and picks up a little cardboard box ("a bag") and a piece of cloth ("a blanket"). She places the bag and the blanket on the "horseback" and says, "now I need food". She picks up some little stones and puts them inside the box. She is straddling "the horse", shouting "Go!" and begins "galloping".

Dana is saying, "Let's pretend you are a baby-mommy. You are a queen, but you are a baby queen, and all this is your nursery." While saying this, Dana is sweeping the whole playground with a grand arm gesture. Ruttie's response is, "Let's pretend I didn't come to the nursery today." She is increasing the tempo of her leg movements.

Dana picks some pieces of plastic out of the junk case, holds them out to Ruttie and says, "Darling, I brought you some food."

Ruttie is responding, "I have a lot of food in my bag" and resumes her galloping.

Dana says, "You should say 'stop', not just 'Go!' all the time."

Ruttie ignored her and continues "galloping". She declares, "At last I've arrived at the village! That's wonderful! I've arrived at the village!"

"Let's pretend we both lived together in that village," Dana is saying.

Ruttie responds, "No, you lived at home and the village was far far away and I lived in it alone."

A macroscopic analysis of the pragmatic level of a play sample like Easy Riders includes the following stages:

(a) Dividing the observed play of each participant in the play interaction into structures, that is, sequences of semantically interpreted activity units that convey specific interpersonal messages.
(b) Formulating the presuppositions of the creator of the structure, regarding the intent or purpose of the other participant.
(c) Formulating the communication purposes of the creator of the structure, based on his or her presuppositions. The presuppositions and purposes apply to the play interaction between two participants only, even if there are more than two participants in the play interaction.

Steps (a) to (c) have been discussed in Chapter 5. Step (d) goes one step further toward a macroscopic analysis.

(d) Determining the proximity/control goals of each of the two participants in relation to the other participant. This stage is based on the assumption that the sequence of presuppositions and purposes associated with each individual structure constitutes a step toward final proximity/control goals.
(e) Classifying the concrete metaphorical images (on the semantic level) of proximity and control created by each of the participants.
(f) Classifying the tactical means, by which each of the two participants attempts to achieve his or her proximity/control goals.

(g) Formulating the strategic plan designed (not necessarily consciously) by each of the two participants for the purpose of reaching his or her proximity/control goals. The strategic plan can be formulated as a set of information-processing programs.

Let us see how such a macroscopic analysis can be applied to Easy Riders.

Steps (a), (b) and (c): Here is a sample of structures in Dana and Ruttie's play, with their presuppositions and purposes.

Dana's structure 1:
Dana calls, "Halt!" and stops moving her legs, looking at Ruttie and making an inviting gesture with an arm.

Presupposition: Ruttie ("the baby" in our play) still has not accepted my invitation to ride with me on horseback, because I was riding alone and have not made a clear invitation gesture.

Purpose: To have Ruttie ride on the horse with me, by stopping the horse and making an unambiguous invitation gesture.

Ruttie's structure 1:
Mounting the horse, sitting in front of Dana, saying, "Let's pretend the baby is in front and the mommy is behind."

Presupposition: Dana wants me to sit on the horse close to her and behind her, she wants to take the lead.

Purpose: To accept Dana's invitation to sit close to her, but to take the lead instead of Dana, on the pretext that a baby sits in front of her mother, who is supposed to protect her from falling.

Ruttie's structure 2:
Calling out "Go!" and start galloping, saying, "Let's pretend the mommy allowed her baby to get lost, because she had a dog. When babies get lost, the dog brings them back. Come on, you got home and told your baby, 'Cutie, you are allowed to get lost.'"

Presuppositions: Dana did not protest my sitting on the horse in front of her, but she wanted to stay on horseback and have me sit close to her.

Purpose: To get Dana off the horse and ride alone, without demanding to stop playing the role of the baby and to provide a convincing justification for my wish to ride alone.

Dana's structure 2:
"Let's pretend you were a baby-mommy, a baby-queen, and all this (the whole playground) is your nursery."

Presupposition: Ruttie wants to ride alone and does not want me to take the lead.

Purposes: To acknowledge and respect Ruttie's dominance and wish to be alone, by letting her be "a mommy" and "a queen", but at the same time not to give up entirely my control position, by partly preserving her role as a "baby" and keeping her in a territory that we share, as it were, by defining the whole playground as "a nursery".

Ruttie's structure 3:
"Let's pretend I didn't come to the nursery today."

Presupposition: Dana wants to remain in a territory that we share.
Purpose: To refuse to remain in a territory shared by Dana, without challenging her role as a mommy-baby or a queen-baby, or the definition of the playground as "a nursery".

Ruttie's structure 4:
"No, you lived at home and the village was far far away and I lived in it alone."

Presupposition: Dana still wants to share with me the same territory.
Purpose: To convey the message that we can't share the same territory and I want to be alone.

(d) An examination of the sequences of presuppositions and purposes associated with each of the structures created by Dana and Ruttie shows quite clearly that Dana's goals are to achieve maximum proximity to Ruttie and to be in a position of control over her, whereas Ruttie's goals are to maintain a maximal distance from Dana and not to allow Dana to control her.

(e) At the raw material level, there is really almost no physical distance between Dana and Ruttie during the play and none of them really controls the other. The struggle for proximity and control between them is conducted at the semantic level, at the level of the symbolic contents of the play. The notions of proximity and control are abstract concepts pertaining to various aspects of interpersonal relations. Children translate these concepts into concrete make-believe play images such as "sitting in front of the horse", "getting off the horse" and "living alone in a distance village".

The concrete, semantic level images of proximity and control in Dana and Ruttie's play can be classified into the following types and subtypes:

Proximity images

Territories
("horseback", "home", "nursery", "village").
Degrees of territorial participation
High participation ("mounting the horse together", "riding together", "living together in the same village").

Medium participation ("stopping the horse", "getting off the horse", "going home", "queen-baby in nursery", "allowed to get lost" and "the dog will bring back").
Low participation ("galloping away", "getting lost", "providing oneself, unaided, with supplies for a long journey", and "living alone in a distant village").

Control images

Controlling roles
("mommy", "queen" and "horse leader").
Controlled roles
("baby" and "back rider").
Controlling activities
("sitting in front", "allowing" and "getting the baby back home").
Controlled activities
("sitting behind", and "be in the nursery").
No control, independence
("galloping", "not coming to the nursery" and "living alone in a distant village").

(f) The tactical tricks conjured up by Dana and Ruttie to achieve their proximity/control goals can be classified into the following types:

A pair of opposites

"mommy-baby". One member of the pair ("mommy") suits Dana's proximity/control goals and the other ("baby") suits Ruttie's.

Drawing a rabbit out of a hat

"The mommy allows her baby to get lost, because she has a dog." Ruttie created, out of void, a dog, in order to soften Dana's resistance to her proximity goal.

Swallowing

"All this is your nursery." The image of an all-embracing nursery "swallowed" Ruttie's attempt to leave their common territory.

Cancelling

"Let's pretend I didn't come to the nursery today." Ruttie cancelled Dana's suggestion, "All this is your nursery."

(g) Here are Dana's and Ruttie's strategic plans for reaching their proximity-control goals:

Dana's plan:

If Ruttie is in *a medium degree of territorial participation*, then I assume *a controlling role* or start *a controlling activity* and invite her to enter my territory, in order to achieve a *high degree of territorial participation*.
If Ruttie resists being in a *controlled role* or resists being engaged in *a controlled activity*, then I sacrifice my *controlling role* or my *controlling activity* but do everything in my capacity to prevent her from going from a *high to medium* and from a *medium to low degree of territorial participation*.

Ruttie's plan:

If Dana is in *a controlling role* or is engaged in *a controlling activity*, then I assume *a controlled role* or enter into *a controlled activity*, but only for a short while. Afterwards I take over her *controlling role* and engage myself in *a controlling activity*. Having accomplished that, I gradually increase the distance between us, moving *from high to medium* and then to *low degree of territorial participation*.
If Dana is not in *a controlling role or activity*, I immediately strive toward *a low degree of territorial participation*.

It will be noted that never in the course of the play Dana and Ruttie confronted one another directly or slipped from managing their conflict in the world of imagination to an open struggle in the real world.

The strategic plan can also be formulated in more detail in information-processing terms, as follows:

Ruttie's plan:

If the input from Dana is "mommy" or "horse leader", "inviting me to join her in riding on the horseback" or "sitting in front of the horseback", I interpret these in my internal processing as attempts to control me.
Then my output is "agreeing to be a baby", "climbing on the horseback" or "getting me, as a baby, back home by the dog", letting her temporarily control me.
Then, if there is no controlling input from Dana, I interpret this in my internal processing as a green light to take control and increase the distance between us. My output is then "sitting in front, being the horse leader", "telling her to allow me to get lost", "galloping" and "preparing for a long-distance ride".
If the further input from Dana is "letting me be a mommy-queen but also a baby", "keeping me in a nursery" or "suggesting that we live together in the distant village", then I interpret this in my internal processing as attempts to control me and prevent me from increasing the distance between us and be alone. My output is then "not coming to the nursery" and "not letting her to live with me together in the distant village".

Interdisciplinary seminar

Lailah: What is the play-therapeutic uses of such macroscopic pragmatic analysis?

Shlomo: As with CDCA, first – understanding the players' language and being able to communicate with them in this language. Second – gaining a deeper understanding of their inter-relationships. Third – helping solve conflicts in group or family play therapy, by transferring the conflicts into the world of make-believe. Fourth – locating bugs in the participants' plans to reach their goals and fix the bugs.

Bugged plans to reach proximity/ control goals are not restricted to make-believe play. Consider for instance the following example:

Husband's proximity goal:
    To get an implicitly defined level of closeness (attention) from wife.
    Husband's plan:
    General presupposition: Wife meets my goal only if I act miserable.

(a) If wife doesn't meet my goal (input), I'll act more miserably (output).
(b) If she does meet my goal (input), I'll just continue being as miserable as before.

Wife's control goal:
    Be dominated by husband, fulfill his wishes.
    Wife's plan:

(a) If my husband's behavior (input) is interpreted by me as having the purpose of needing help (internal processing), then I act according to my control goal and extend help (output).
(b) If his behavior (input) is interpreted by me as an indication that he doesn't have the purpose of getting help (internal processing), then I act according to my goal and withdraw help (output).
(c) If my husband continues being miserable despite help (input), then I interpret this as an indication that he doesn't have the purpose of getting help (internal processing).

Go back to (a).

You can see that both the husband's and the wife's plans are bugged. The bugs guarantee that none of them, especially the husband, will ever reach their goals.

Ethan: Let me try to specify the bugs. The husband's general hypotheses, "wife meets my goal only if I act miserable" is wrong, non-sense. It is also horse blindered because he has no clue about his wife's goal to please him, to fulfil his wishes.

Lailah: It is also infected with fifth wheel, because his acting miserable is irrelevant to their real goals, which are complementary. But it is not infected with flip-flop, because it is consistent.

Anna: The wife's plan is also infected with both non-sense and horse blinders, because she does not process the information that her husband's goal is not to get help but to get attention.
Shlomo: Excellent!

Summary of chapter 7

Relations between human (and non-human) individuals and groups revolve around the parameters of proximity and control. Macroscopic pragmatic analysis of group or family make-believe play is a heuristic procedure for exposing the proximity-control goals of the participants and their strategic plans to reach their goals. The steps of such a macroscopic analysis are (a) dividing the observed play of each participant in the play interaction into structures; (b) formulating the presuppositions of the creator of the structure, as to the intent or purpose of the other participant; (c) formulating the communication purpose of the creator of the structure; (d) determining the proximity/control goals of each of the two participants with respect to the other participant; (e) classifying the concrete metaphorical images (on the semantic level) of proximity and control created by each of the participants; (f) classifying the tactical means by which each of the two participants attempts to achieve his or her proximity/control goals; (g) Formulating the strategic plan designed by each of the two participants for the purpose of reaching his or her proximity/control goals. The strategic plan can be formulated as a set of information-processing programs; and (h) detecting bugs in the strategic plans.

One of the advantages of group or family make-believe play is the possibility of transferring proximity-control conflicts into the imaginative world of make-believe. The bugs in the strategic plans can be weakened or removed by play bug-busters.

Assignments

1. Do a complete macroscopic pragmatic analysis of the following observation of a family's make-believe play, using the concepts and techniques introduced in this chapter. Identify and name the bugs in the plans for reaching the proximity-control goals of each of the participants:

Observation 7.2 Sara, Gabby and Maayan
Sara, a single parent, with her seven-year-old son Gabby and her eight-year-old daughter Maayan.

Maayan: I am the princess and Mommy is the queen.
   She gives her mother a toy crown and covers her shoulders with a gold-colored cloth that she found in the costumes box. She moves a

> low chair to the chair on which Sara is sitting and sits down on the low chair with her head resting on Sara's shoulder.
>
> Gabby is standing away from Sara and Maayan. He wears a policeman's hat and holds a toy gun.
>
> *Gabby*: I am a wanted criminal disguised as a cop. You don't know I'm a criminal. I told the queen to help us, the police, catch the criminal, but if she does not want to help, I'll take you both as hostages.
>
> *Maayan*: Mother queen, do you know this cop? He doesn't look to me like a real cop.
>
> *Sara*: I know all the cops in my kingdom. He is not a real cop. I'll call my servants and they will handcuff him and put him in the dungeon of the palace.
>
> Gabby puts on a clown mask and says, "I just was fooling you. I am the queen's clown."
>
> *Maayan*: Mother-queen, don't believe him. He is not the real clown. He is the criminal.
>
> Gabby takes a demon doll and says in a "demonic" voice, "I'm not a criminal at all, not a cop or a clown. I'm a demon from hell and I'm going to turn you into dolls and take you to hell and burn you!"
>
> He is running toward Sara and Maayan, howling, and hits Maayan's arm with the demon doll.
>
> *Sara*: Gabby, stop it!

A classified list of publications

Pragmatics

Huang, Y. (2015). *Pragmatics*. Oxford, UK: Oxford University Press.

Pragmatic analysis of play observations

Ariel, S. (1992). *Strategic family play therapy*. Chichester, UK: Wiley.
Ariel, S. (1997). *Culturally competent family therapy*. Westport, CT: Praeger.
Ariel, S. (2002). *Children's imaginative play: A visit to Wonderland*. Westport, CT: Praeger.
Ariel, S. (2018). *Multi-dimensional therapy with families, children and adults: The Diamond Model*. London, UK: Routledge.

Part 3

The manifold magic of make-believe play

Chapter 8
A formal definition of make-believe play

In Chapter 2, Rudolf Carnap's concept of *explication* is mentioned. Carnap defined *explication* as the replacement of a vague pre-scientific concept with a well-defined concept. It was argued that it is impossible to explicate, in this sense, the cover term *play*, but that it is possible to define the concept of *make-believe play* in a formal and precise manner. Such an explicit definition has far-reaching implications with respect to therapeutic applications of make-believe play.

Make-believe play is primarily a mental activity, whose outward manifestations are verbal, non-verbal or both. This mental activity comprises the following mental operations, performed simultaneously:

Realification of a purely mental entity. The player implicitly or explicitly tells himself /herself that a mental entity in his/her mind is present in the immediate external environment at the very time of the play, not as a mental entity but as a concrete, tangible, perceptible entity. e.g. "The image of a lion in my mind is a real lion, actually present in the immediate external environment here and now."

The realified mental entities can be a single image of a real or imaginary creature or object (e.g. a cookie monster, a car), a class of such images (e.g. Pokémon, trains), properties of such classes (e.g. "the bad ones", "inflating monsters"), relations between such classes (e.g. "the bad ones vs. the good ones"), or propositions standing for real, possible, hypothetical, nonsensical or imaginary individuals, properties and states of affairs (e.g. "Mommy is changing the baby's diaper"; "The Jumblies went to sea in a sieve."). In the player's mind, the realified mental entity exists in specified or unspecified, real or imaginary time and place.

The realification can be verbalized, (e.g. saying "There is a lion here now"; "The bad ones are chasing the good ones") and/or signified by some concrete entity present or created by the player in the immediate environment – a toy, a piece of paper, the player's body, the player's voice, etc. For example, the player produces a roaring sound to signify the realified lion or signifies the realified lion by a clothes peg.

Moreover, the player *identicates* the *signifier* (i.e. the entity that signifies the realified image) with the *signified* (i.e. the realified entity). *Identication* means that the entity chosen to signify the realified mental image is no longer taken to be what it usually is, but has actually been transformed into the realified mental image (e.g. the player's voice is no longer taken to be his or her own voice but an actual lion's roar, or the clothing peg is no longer considered a clothing peg but the realified lion).

The actual time and place of playing are also identicated. A boy is blowing a balloon in his nursery at four in the afternoon and is making-believe that the balloon is an inflatable monster existing in some unspecified time and place. Then the boy's room is being identicated with that unspecified time and place. It is no longer his own room but the realified place in which the inflatable monster is present. The time of playing is also identicated. It is no longer four in the afternoon but the realified unspecified time in which the inflatable monster is present.

The third mental operation is *denial of seriousness*. It is a meta-operation, a mental operation about the above two mental operations. The player does not believe that a real lion is actually present in the immediate environment at the time of playing, nor does he believe that his own voice is a lion's roar or that the clothing peg is not a clothing peg but a lion. He does not really believe that his nursery is not his nursery but the unspecified place in which an inflatable monster is present, nor does he believe that the time of playing, four in the afternoon, is not really the time of playing but the unspecified time in which the inflatable monster is present. He is making these mental claims just for the fun of it.

To summarize: Make-believe play is defined as the simultaneous activation of the mental claims *realification* (which can be verbalized) *identication* and *denial of seriousness*.

This definition covers all and only the phenomena constituting make-believe play properly so-called. It draws clear distinctions between make-believe play and akin, superficially similar phenomena such as, fantasy and imagination, deferred imitation, symbolic representation, errors of identification, delusions, hallucinations, dreams, attempts to mislead, storytelling, drama and rituals.

Fantasy, imagination, daydreams. As mentioned above, realified mental entities can include fictional beings, objects and situations. They will not be considered make-believe play, unless they are realifed by being verbalized and/or signified by identicated concrete entities that have been created or chosen by the player at the very time and place of play. Moreover, they will not be considered make-believe play unless the actual playing time and place are identicated with the realified time and place as well. And they will not be considered make-believe play unless the seriousness of the realification and identication are implicitly or explicitly denied.

Deferred imitation. Imagine a girl mimicking the sounds and movements of a monkey. On the face of it this looks like make-believe play. It is not. There is no realification. The girl is not pretending that a real monkey is present in the immediate external environment of the play at the time of the play. There is no identication either. The girl is not pretending that she is not herself but the realified monkey.

Symbolic representation. A boy is making a sand palace on the beach. It is a symbolic representation of a palace. However, it is not an instance of make-believe play. The boy is not pretending that the sand structure is not a sand structure but a real palace. No realification and no identication.

Error of identification, a misperception or miscategorization. A girl sees a toy apple and believes it is a real apple. She is trying to eat it. This is not make-believe play, because there is no denial of seriousness. A toddler does not yet know the difference between a dog and a donkey. He sees a donkey and says "doggie". This is not make-believe play because there is no denial of seriousness.

Hallucination. One should distinguish between a hallucination that is a kind of misperception and a hallucination in which ones sees or hears something that does not exist in a tangible way in the immediate external environment. An example of a hallucination of the first kind: A person sees his roommate holding a pomegranate and "sees" a grenade. This is not just a misperception or a miscategorization, because it is a projection based on the linguistic similarity between the two objects. An example of a hallucination of the second kind: A person hears a voice telling him that his roommate is plotting to kill him. Both kinds of hallucination are not make-believe play, because there is no denial of seriousness.

Delusion. A girl claims and believes she is a real fairy. This is not make-believe play because there is no denial of seriousness.

A dream. A person is dreaming that he is being transformed into a monster. This is not make-believe play, because there is no denial of seriousness. Furthermore, there is no realification, because in a dream there is no separation between mental reality and external reality. The dreamer believes that the internal reality is external reality. The same applies to hallucinations and delusions.

Storytelling is not make-believe play, even if the story is being told in the present tense, because there is no realification and no identication. Suppose the storyteller is saying, "Sam is playing with his little dinosaur." If the storyteller does not pretend that Sam and his dinosaur are actually present in the storyteller's immediate external environment at the time of playing, this is not make-believe play. The time and place of the storytelling are not identicated with the imaginary time and place of the story's content.

An attempt to mislead. A girl is trying to convince a boy that she is a real princess. This is not make-believe play. The denial of seriousness is not an attempt to mislead or cheat. It is made just for the fun of it. If a player shares his or her make-believe play, both parties know that it is just make-believe play.

Drama. Although on the face of it dramatic acts seem to be identical to make-believe play, they are not. The definition of make-believe play proposed here specifies the necessary and sufficient conditions for an activity to be qualified as make-believe play. Drama fulfills the necessary but not the sufficient conditions, e.g. reciting a play or a script, the semi-ritualized and conventionalized nature of the occasion and the presence of audience.

Improvised drama. This kind of activity seems to have all the necessary and sufficient conditions to be qualified as make-believe play. It is however in most cases not a spontaneous activity like children's make-believe play, but a ritualized and conventionalized activity in which the participants follow some instructions, e.g. asked to improvise on a given theme.

Ritual. Certain rituals appear to be similar to make-believe play, e.g. the Naven ceremony of a New Guinea tribe, in which a male pretends to be a pregnant woman (Bettelheim 1955, p. 2). It will require a special sort of anthropological research to determine what kinds of mental claims are implicitly made in the framework of such rituals. At any rate, it is quite clear that they are different from make-believe play in a number of respects. Unlike make-believe play, a ritual is stereotyped, bound to specific contexts, totally learned and scripted and serves various functions beyond itself.

The term *play bug-busters*, introduced in Chapter 3, refers to those curative properties of make-believe play that can serve as techniques for removing or weakening bugs in programs that belong to internal or external subsystems. The following play bug-busters can be logically derived from the above formal definition of the concept make-believe play.

Owning and alienation. In make-believe play the player both owns and disowns the semantic contents of his or her play.

The owning is logically derived from the mental claims of realification and identication. Imagine for instance a boy aiming a toy gun at his playmate, saying, "I'm killing you." The mental claims of realification and identication imply the player owns the acts of shooting and killing. In other words, both his verbal and non-verbal expressions imply that he is not really a boy playing with his playmate, but a real gunman shooting a real victim at the very place and time in which these expressions are being uttered and performed. These place and time are however identicated with the imaginary place and time in which the shooting occurs. The mental claim *denial of seriousness* implies the player also *disowns* the contents of his play, *alienates* himself from it. In the above example, for instance, the player's verbal and non-verbal acts imply, "I don't really believe that I am a real gunman shooting my victim with a real gun here and now. I am just a boy playing with my playmate and am pretending to be a real shooter just for the fun of it."

Needless to say, the owning and alienation property of make-believe play is a priceless gift for children, because it enables them to express forbidden wishes, e.g. to get rid of a newborn sibling, to engage in prohibited activities such as violence and aggression, to fearlessly face scary creatures such as monsters, and so forth. In play therapy, the therapist can help activate this property as a means of getting rid of or weaken bugs.

Basic duality. In make-believe play the player is both his or her own real-self, present in the play's real time and location, and a character in his or her make-believe play, an insider who is present in the imaginary make-believe time and location. The person making the mental claims of realification and identication is the player, a real person in real specific time and place. By making these two claims the player transfers himself or herself to the realm of make-believe. However, the player is also the real person who is making the mental claim of denial of seriousness. This meta claim implies that he is his real-self, not in the realm of make-believe but in the real-world at the time and place of playing. In the above example of the boy aiming a toy gun at his playmate, saying, "I'm killing you", the player is both his real-self and the character in his play.

Arbitrariness of the signifier. The signifier is a raw material entity that is identicated with the realified signified. The latter belongs to the semantic level. The signifier is arbitrary in the sense that any tangible entity whatsoever can signify any realified content. For example, a girl plays as if a creature called Pampy is swallowing itself. Pampy is signified (identicated) in her play by a paper bag that she has turned inside out.

Possible worlds. In make-believe play any past, present or future, realistic, imaginary or absurd event or situation can be created by the player without restriction. The above example of the girl playing as if a creature called Pampy is swallowing itself illustrates this property too.

Interdisciplinary seminar

Shlomo: Let's go back to Case 1.1 (Rusella) that we discussed in our first session. Let's see how owing and alienation can be activated as a means of getting rid of horse blinders and non-sense.

In case 1.1 (Rusella) it was narrated that Rusella's mother and her 14-year-old brother were mimicking her awkward way of walking and her baby talk. They found it funny. While in school Rusella would respond to the harassment with blows and kicks, at home she would join her mother and brother's laughter when they imitated her, so they saw it as an amusing game that Rusella enjoyed too.

This abusive interaction can be seen as part of the proximity plan between Rusella and her mother and brother. Her mother and brother's plan was tainted with horse blinders and non-sense. They misinterpreted her compliance, didn't realize how hurt she was and didn't understand why she co-operated. Russella's co-operation was infected with horse blinders, because she didn't consider other ways of getting proximity, without letting them make fun of her.

A therapist could try to help Rusella, her mother and her brother to get rid of these bugs by a conversation, in which both sides, mediated by the therapist, explain themselves and add missing data. I'm not sure it would work. Apparently, it wouldn't be easy for Rusella to speak openly and explain herself. Her mother and brother would probably feel criticized and attacked. Play therapy in which owning and alienation were activated would make it easier, emotionally and cognitively, to expose and weaken these bugs.

Let's see first how owning and alienation can be activated in individual therapy with Rusella.

I am reading a part of Lailah's description of her session with Rusella (Session 1.1). A suitable moment to enter Rusella's play and make a move would seem to be the point at which she introduced her relationship with her mother into the play:

> "She got up and brought a woman doll, a girl doll and a baby doll. She approached me, turned in my direction, handed over to me the woman doll and said, "The mother told the girl to take care of the baby and the girl didn't want to. Then the mother sent the girl alone to the forest."

Can you think of an idea how to join the play and activate owning and alienation?

Ethan: I don't see how. You said that Rusella's co-operation with her mother and brother's derisive imitation of her way of speaking and walking was part of her plan to achieve a rapport with her mother and brother. But in this play episode she wasn't trying to achieve closeness. She was rebelling against her mother's attempt to control her.

Shlomo: Do you remember the play of the two girls, Dana and Ruttie? (Observation 7.1). This is an example of how it is possible to struggle both for control and for proximity through make-believe play.

Anna: At this point I would suggest to Rusella to tell her mother, "I will take care of the baby only if you do not laugh at my walking and talking and play with me nicely." This would lift the horse blinders because it would help Rusella to be aware that she feels exploited, hurt by her mother's mockery and wants a positive closeness. It would also help Rusella understand that she should communicate this message openly to her mother.

Daniel: But this is not playful. It is a direct message.

Anna: Why? I mean that the girl in the play, the doll, would tell this to the mother in the play, also a doll.

Shlomo: Still, it sounds like a direct message rather than play.

I have an idea. Rusella gave you a woman doll and asked you to "be" the mother. I'd stay in the role of the mother but assume an additional role. Previously, Rusella introduced into her play a large teddy-bear character, who protected the rabbit from the gorilla. So, Rusella would probably be willing to admit me to her play in the role of the teddy-bear too.

Lailah, let's role-play it. You'll be Rusella and I'll be therapist. Get a woman doll, a girl doll and a baby doll. Hand the woman doll over to me and ask me to be the mother.

I get the teddy-bear doll and hold it in my right hand. I hold the mother doll in my left hand.

I whisper to the ear of the girl doll that's held by Lailah (in the role of Rusella), "Your mother can't see or hear me, only you can. I'm going to hide the baby doll behind my back."

I take the baby doll (representing Rusella's little sister) from Lailah and hide it behind the teddy-bear's back.

Then, as the bear, I tell the girl doll (representing Rusella), "Let's pretend that you played as if you were the baby, walking like a baby and talking like a baby. Your mom will think you are the baby, not the older sister."

I tell Lailah, "Lailah, I'm not sure Rusella would comply, but for the sake of the role play, please do it."

Lailah makes the girl doll walk and talk like a baby.

I make the mother doll laugh goodheartedly and say, "What a cute baby I have! I love to see how she is toddling and stumbling, and I enjoy her babbling and baby-talk so much! But where is my girl, her older sister? She disappeared! I'm busy. She should take care of her little sister."

I, with a big smile, make the teddy-bear whisper to the girl doll that's held in Lailah's hand, "Your mom really believed you were the baby and not the older sister, but now your mom will be able to see and hear me too."

I make the teddy-bear that's held in my right hand say to the woman's doll that's held in my left hand, "Hi, I'm the bear with very little brain. Do you have any honey for me?"

I answer as the mother, "No, no, I have no honey."

Then I'd say in a silly bear's voice, pointing at the girl doll, "You thought she was the baby, right? She wasn't the baby, she was the big sister. She just pretended to be the baby."

I make the mother ask me, as the teddy-bear, "Is that right? Why did she pretend to be the baby?"

I, as the teddy-bear, tell the mother doll, "You can have three guesses. If you are right, she, the older sister, will nod. If you are wrong, she'll turn her head from side to side."

Then, as the mother, I say to the girl's doll, "First guess: Because you wanted me to breast-feed you."

Lailah makes the girl doll turn her head from side to side.

I say, as the mother doll, "Second guess: Because you wanted me to change your diapers."

Lailah turns her head from side to side.

I make the mother doll say, "Third guess: Because you wanted me to tell you what I said when I thought you were the baby, that you are cute and all these nice things."

Lailah makes the girl doll nod.

Then, as the teddy-bear, I tell the mother doll, "I'm a silly bear with very little brain. I'm hungry and you refused to give me honey, so at least I want you to tell me sweet thing."

I make the teddy-bear toddle and stumble and babble like a baby.

I, as the bear, tell the mother doll, "Why aren't you saying how cute I am?"

Then I make the mother laugh and imitate my movements in a mocking way.

I say, as the mother doll "Because you are funny, you are a big silly bear with very little brain, pretending to be a baby."

I laugh and whisper to the girl doll that's held in Lailah's hand, "You know why I am laughing? Because I don't want your mother to know that what she said made me sad and angry."

Shlomo: Lailah, how was this role play for you?
Lailah: I don't know, a bit confusing. I tried to put myself in Rusella's shoes. It did do something powerful to me emotionally, but during the role play I was unable to analyze what was happening to me.
Shlomo: Your responses are typical of the experience that clients undergo when play bug-busters are activated. Such an experience is present in the twilight

zone between emotion and insight. The play bug-busters have their therapeutic power precisely because they immediately get the clients into such a mental–emotional state.

Lailah: Your last statement, "I don't want your mother to know that what she said made me sad and angry." It was too direct for me, not sufficiently disguised by the owning and alienation of play. It made me upset.

Shlomo: A good lesson for me and us.

Anna: That was quite directive, more like a show than like an interactive play.

Daniel: You were quite playful and funny and seemed to be able to communicate with the girl in her own play language. Although you were directive, you didn't impose anything. You played the role of the mother because Rusella asked you to play this role. You chose the teddy-bear because Rusella introduced the teddy-bear into the play as a protective agent. And you seemed to be flexible, playing two roles at the same time, changing roles and characters, etc. This is a method of doing play therapy I would like to assimilate.

Ethan: Let me see if I understand how you activated the owning and alienation in your intervention. What kind of bugs you wanted to bust by your play bug-busters?

Daniel: The way I see it, the bug is horse blinders. Rusella wasn't aware, or wasn't fully aware, that her baby-talk at home was a part of her plan to get proximity to her mother, to enlist her mother's positive attention and expressions of love. She wanted her mother to show that she was enjoying her company. Rusella also wasn't fully aware that by behaving like a baby she did not get positive attention, but negative and offensive, because she was ridiculous rather than cute.

Lailah: She also wasn't fully aware how hurt she was when her mother and brother imitated her. She wasn't in touch with the realization that her laughter was meant to hide her insult and anger. Your involvement in the play was designed to remove the horse blinders and increase her awareness of all of these. But as I said, at some point you were too direct.

Shlomo: My purpose was to help her be in touch with the relevant information, not just cognitively but also emotionally, to verbalize her thoughts and emotions, give them shape.

Ethan: Your main interventions were: Making the girl doll behave like a baby; presenting the mother as enjoying the baby's behavior, but not the bear's pretending to be a baby; saying clearly that the bear was laughing to hide his having been hurt and angry.

Shlomo: How was the owning and alienation activated to achieve all these?

Daniel: First, all your messages were introduced not directly but through make-believe figures in a make-believe time and place. I think this is an application not just of owning and alienation but also of basic duality, because you were both the mother and the teddy-bear and yourself, Shlomo, the play therapist. The girl doll and the baby doll were both make-believe figures and the real Rusella. The mother doll was both a make-believe figure and Rusella's real mother. So Rusella knew in a way that it was all about her relationship with her mother and about you as a therapist.

Ethan: You said, as the teddy-bear, not directly to Rusella, but to her girl doll, "Let's pretend that you play as if you are the baby, walking like a baby and talking like a baby. Your mom will think you are the baby, not the older sister." It looks like delving into deeper and deeper layers of make-believe, make-believe within make-believe within make-believe, reinforcing the alienation aspect of the play. First you pretended that you were the teddy-bear and Rusella was a make-believe girl. Then you, as the teddy-bear, told the make-believe girl to pretend that she play as if she were the baby. Then you told the girl that her mother would be misled by the make-believe act, which is nonsense, another form of make-believe. Although the owning aspect is there too, I think Rusella could be fascinated by the opportunity to dive deeply into the make-believe world.

Anna: I like the idea that you, as the teddy-bear, behaved like a baby and exposed yourself to the mother's ridicule. Instead of exposing the girl to this insult, you exposed yourself and modeled for Rusella. You used lots of "as ifs", of pretending, like laughing, pretending to enjoy when you were really hurt and angry.

Shlomo: Let's look at the bug-buster arbitrariness of the signifier. Here is an example of activating arbitrariness of the signifier to bust the bug flip-flop in the control plan of a father with respect to his nine-year-old son. The father, using strict methods of education, imposed iron-discipline on his son. The boy used to beat up his younger brother. His father punished him by beating him up, saying, "I'm beating him up to teach him not to beat up his brother." This control plan is infected with flip-flop, a self-contradiction.

In a family play therapy, the family played as if the parents took their two sons to have a good time at the mall. The therapist played as if she were a waitress in a restaurant where the family had lunch. During the imaginary meal, the father repeatedly told the boy that he should sit nicely and eat politely. The therapist, as the waitress, came with a cart and said to the father, "We have a children's meal here. Let the boy choose what you think he needs to eat. Come and see what we have here for children's dinner: A bagel with a very nutritious spread."

She shows the father a toy snake curled into a circle. She says, "Here is a spinach pie. It makes the boy grow fast and strong." She shows the father a boxing glove.

Can you analyze this intervention?

Lailah: I can see the arbitrariness of the signifier here. The snake is an arbitrary signifier on the raw material level for the content "a nutritious bagel" on the semantic level. The boxing glove on the raw material level is an arbitrary signifier for the spinach pie on the semantic level. It reminds me of Popeye the Sailor. Here too I see a make-believe within make-believe. The therapist makes believe as if she is the waitress, and as a waitress she makes believe as if the snake is a bagel and the boxing glove is a spinach pie. The make-believe waitress realifies the ideas of a bagel and a spinach pie and identicates the toy snake and the boxing glove with the realified bagel and spinach pie.

Anna: There is a contradiction between the aggressive connotations of the snake and boxing glove as signifiers and the benevolent connotations of the signified – nutrition, strengthening. I think this hints at the contradiction between the father's wish to edify his son not to be violent or misbehave and the father's violent and harsh disciplinary and controlling methods. So, the arbitrariness of the signifier here is a bug-buster, busting the bug flip-flop by indirectly exposing the contradiction.

Shlomo: Good!

Daniel: I have two questions. First, would the father understand this message? Second, if he does, wouldn't he feel criticized and attacked?

Shlomo: From my experience, there is no need to be too explicit in using the bug-busters. Even if the client doesn't figure out exactly what the therapist is trying to say, he somehow feels that there is a message there. So, in a way this message sinks in, even if not fully consciously. As to feeling criticized, yes, especially as this father is harsh and rigid. But hopefully he would take it lightly, thanks to the softening effect of the owning and alienation and the basic duality.

Here is another example of the use of arbitrariness of the signifier as a means of busting the bugs horse blinders and non-sense in the proximity-control plans between mother and daughter.

Session 8.1 Tessa and Kate

Tessa, a divorcee, wanted to send her ten-year-old daughter Kate to a boarding school. Both claimed they were not getting along. Both said that they "get on each other's nerves". The therapist understood their quarrels as reflecting their bugged (horse blindered) plan to overcome their over-dependence on each other. Their mutual proximity-control goals were to separate, to create arbitrary boundaries between them.

In one of the therapeutic sessions, Tessa and Kate played the following scene: Tessa as "a queen" expelled Kate "the princess" to the forest. The therapist played the role of "good fairy". He promised to lead the princess to a hut in the forest where she would be protected. He led her to Tessa, after having asked her to "be" the hut. Kate sat in her lap. Tessa's body, particularly her lap, served as an arbitrary signifier for the signified content "a hut in the forest", hinting at the boarding school.

Shlomo: The contradiction between the physical proximity of the mother and the daughter, the warmth and tenderness of Tessa's lap on the one hand and the cold and distant hut on the other, meant to make Tessa and Kate feel and be aware of the strong emotional bond between them and the difficulty of disengaging from one another. The horse blinders were removed. That opened the way for them to explore more adequate ways for developing mutual autonomy, without turning each other's life into hell and without losing each other.

Anna: Turning the mother's body into an arbitrary signifier for a hut in the forest is an ingenious original idea. But a therapist must be very creative to pull such rabbits out of her hats.

Shlomo: Yes, a play therapist who is an active participant in the clients' play must be creative. But, as I said in one of our previous sessions, everyone can be creative. It is a matter of overcoming inhibitions.

Here is an example of busting the bugs fifth-wheel and horse blinders.

Session 8.2 Sofia

The bug was in the body image program of a 12-year-old girl, Sofia. Till the age of 11 she had been overweight and clumsy. She suffered from social rejection. During her 12th year her physique was changing dramatically as a result of dieting, exercise and natural maturation processes. She looked good, dressed well, played tennis and danced and became popular in the company of her peers. But she couldn't get rid of her previous self and body image. A part of her still saw herself as fat, ugly and clumsy. Her body image was infected with fifth wheel, because the previous state of her body and her social status were completely irrelevant to her current situation. Her therapist, who herself was thin and shapely, suggested that both of them play as if they were plus-size models. The therapist had a whole assortment of used costumes. She brought dresses and clothes that were several sizes big on their bodies. Both dressed (over their clothes, of course) before a mirror and then they walked clumsily on a pretend runway, almost falling.

The therapist placed large dolls on both sides of the runway, as an audience, playing as if they were shouting, "Where did you get such fat and ugly models?!"

The therapist whispered to the girl on the runway, "Don't pay attention to them, it's their problem, not ours. We are beautiful as we are."

Sofia enjoyed this play very much and was laughing continuously. At the next session they played as if they were top models dressed in elegant, slim clothes. The therapist made the audience yell contemptuously, "We don't want such thin models!" Sofia, spontaneously, shouted, "Shut up, we are beautiful as we are!"

Anna: I think in both sessions the bug-buster that was activated was possible worlds.

Lailah: Owning and alienation and basic duality too. In the first session, Sofia could actually see in her own eyes that she was not fat, because the big-size clothes emphasized her being slim. She could own her being slim but at the same time be alienated from it, giving room for her fears about her body. In the second session, she could own the memory of the insulting reactions of her peers, but also alienate herself from it.

Anna: I feel a bit uneasy about this play intervention. In recent years there is a lot of talk about the cult of thinness and beauty, about anorexic models. In this play the therapist seems to encourage the girl to attribute excessive importance to external beauty.

Ethan: But this is therapy, Anna, not ideological preaching.

Lailah: I am not sure I agree with you, Anna. It seems to me that while helping Sofia get rid of her distorted body image, the therapist actually conveyed through the play the idea that one should not attach too much weight to body weight.

Daniel (smiling): Too much weight, body weight.

Summary of chapter 8

This chapter is devoted to a formal explication of the concept make-believe play and to play-therapeutic corollaries of this explication. Make-believe play is primarily a mental activity, whose outward manifestations are verbal, non-verbal or both. This activity comprises the following mental operations, performed simultaneously: *Realification* of a purely mental entity, implicitly claiming that it is present in the immediate external environment at the very time of the play. The realification can be verbalized or signified by some concrete entity present or created by the player in the immediate environment. The player *identicates* the entity chosen to signify the realified mental entity. *Identication* means that the entity chosen to signify the realified image is no longer taken to be what it usually is but has actually been transformed into the realified mental image. The actual time and place of playing are also identicated with the imaginary time and place of the realified entity. The third mental operation is *denial of seriousness*. It is a meta-operation, denying the seriousness or validity of the realification and identication. This definition covers all the phenomena constituting make-believe play. It draws clear distinctions between make-believe play and akin, superficially similar phenomena such as fantasy and imagination, deferred imitation, symbolic representation, errors of identification, delusions, hallucinations, dreams, attempts to mislead, storytelling, fantasy and imagination, drama and rituals.

The term *play bug-busters* refer to those curative properties of make-believe play that can serve as techniques for removing or weakening bugs in programs that belong to internal or external subsystems. The following play bug-busters can be logically derived from the above formal definition of the concept make-believe play:

Owning and alienation. In make-believe play, the player both owns and disowns the semantic contents of his or her play. The owning and alienation property of make-believe play enables players to express forbidden wishes, engage in prohibited activities or fearlessly face scary creatures. In play therapy, therapists can help activate this property as a means of getting rid of or weaken bugs. *Basic duality.* In make-believe play the player is both his or her own real self and a character in his or her make-believe play, an insider who is present in the imaginary make-believe time and location. The player can witness his or her own imaginary characters and events as both an insider and an outsider. *Arbitrariness of the signifier.* Any tangible entity whatsoever can signify any realified content. *Possible worlds.* In make-believe play any past, present or future, realistic, imaginary or absurd event or situation can be created by the player without restriction. In play therapy, these bug-buster can be used to lift horse blinders, get rid of fifth wheels, settle flip-flops and correct non-sense.

Assignments

1. Explain in your own words and illustrate your explanations with your own examples:
   Why and how are the bug-busters owning and alienation, basic duality, arbitrariness of the signifier and possible worlds derived logically from the formal definition of make-believe play?
2. Provide your own examples of uses of the bug-busters owing and alienation, basic duality, arbitrariness of the signifier and possible worlds as means for weakening or removing bugs in bugged individual and interpersonal programs.
3. Identify the bugs in the various programs in Case 3.2 (Kabr). Propose ways of activating the play bug-busters owning and alienation, basic duality, arbitrariness of the signifier and possible worlds as a means of weakening or removing the bugs.

A classified list of publications

Definitions of the concept make-believe play

Ariel, S. (2002). *Children's imaginative play: A visit to Wonderland.* Westport, CT: Praeger.

Ariel, S. (2018). *Multi-dimensional therapy with families, children and adults: The Diamond Model.* London, UK: Routledge.

Bateson, G. (1956). The message 'this is play'. In: Schaffner, B., ed. *Group processes: Transactions of the second conference .* New York, NY: Josiah Macy, Jr. Foundation, pp. 145–242.

Piaget, J. (1962). *Play, dreams and imitation in childhood.* New York, NY: Norton.

Winnicott, D. (1971). *Playing and reality.* London, UK: Tavistock.

Bugs in internal and external programs

Ariel, S. (1992). *Strategic family play therapy.* Chichester, UK: Wiley.
Ariel, S. (2018). *Multi-dimensional therapy with families, children and adults: The Diamond Model.* London, UK: Routledge.
Dumas, J.E., Lemay, Ph. and Dauwalder, J.P. (2001). Dynamic analyses of mother-child interactions in functional and dysfunctional dyads: A synergetic approach. *Journal of Abnormal Child Psychology* 29 (4), pp.317–329.
Sullaway, M. and Christensen, A. (1983). Assessment of dysfunctional interaction patterns in couples. *Journal of Marriage and the Family* 45 (3), pp.653–660.

The healing powers of play

Bettelheim, B. (1955). *Truants from life.* New York, NY: Simon and Schuster.
Schaefer, Ch.E. and Drewes, A.A. (2013). *The therapeutic powers of play: 20 core agents of change.* Hoboken, NJ: Wiley.

Chapter 9

Linguistic peculiarities of make-believe play

In Chapter 2, the frequently brought forward argument that young children are incapable of activating verbal meta-cognition (thinking about one's own thinking) is examined critically. It has been stated there that verbal therapy does not suit young children because their command of language and their verbal meta-cognition capacity are still rather limited. That is why play is the preferable medium for child therapy. This statement implies that play is non-verbal and does not allow for meta-cognition. This is incorrect. Many children as young as four or five often use fairly rich verbal language in their play. They are quite sophisticated in their use of language. Furthermore, meta-cognition is an inherent property of make-believe play, because children distinguish between play and non-play and often comment about the contents of their own play. Take for instance the following statement, said by a mother about her little son, "Sometimes I feel that I can't stand him, even hate him. I know that I love him more than anything else in the world and that I am saying this to myself only because he sometimes makes it difficult for me to deal with him." This statement can be qualified as an instance of meta-cognition. But consider the following statement, said by a six-year-old boy to his playmate, "Let's play as if I hate my mother because she loves my brother more than she loves me." Such statements, often made by very young children in their make-believe play, are instances of meta-cognition. The denial of seriousness inherent in make-believe play indicates that the boy knows that he does not really hate his mother. Such make-believe play statements are instances of meta-cognition no less than the above words expressed by the mother.

Let us look at the peculiar characteristics of the use of language in make-believe play and see how these characteristics can be implemented in gainful manners in play therapy.

Some of the linguistic peculiarities of make-believe play derive from its very definition, that is, from the mental claims of realification, identication and denial of seriousness. As asserted in Chapter 8, the actual time and place of playing are also identicated with the realified contents. The player implicitly claims that the very time and place of playing are not really the concrete time and place of playing but the time and place of the realified entity, which can be specified or unspecified. Thus, in the make-believe play of children one hears expressions like "Now is tomorrow", "Now is yesterday", "Now is not now", "Now is then", "Now we are being born", "Here is not here", "Here is there", "It is night time now (said in a daytime)", "Here is the moon" (said in the player's kindergarten). In ordinary language such expressions would be considered self-contradictory or false. But in make-believe play they are not, because, thanks to the denial of seriousness, they are ambiguous. The player implicitly claims that the play does not occur at the immediate environment at the time of playing. But the player also implicitly or explicitly denies the seriousness of this claim. This implies that the play does occur at the actual immediate time and place of playing. An expression such as "Now is tomorrow" therefore means, "Now (the actual time of playing) is not now but tomorrow, but since I am not saying this seriously, I know that now is really the actual time of playing." Likewise, the expression "Here is there" means "Here (the actual location of playing) is not here but there, at an imaginary make-believe place, but since I am not saying this seriously, I know that here is really the actual location of playing."

The use of such peculiar linguistic expressions in make-believe play has various advantages, which can be utilized in play therapy. Such expressions can serve as bug-busters, busting the bugs horse blinders, fifth wheel, flip-flop and non-sense.

Session 9.1 Eli and his mother

Eli (8) would curse his mother and throw things at her when she did not let him do or have what he wanted. He would shout, "You hate me! You don't want me! You want to get rid of me!"

When the tantrum was over, he would calm down, hug his mother, act like an angel and completely forget how he had behaved before. At one of the sessions, he refused to enter the room and when he did come in he went wild, yelled at his mother and began throwing objects at her. She was at a loss. The therapist, Ezra, said, "Let's play as if Mommy is the bad guys and we are the good guys and I am your commander."

Ezra gave the mother and Eli toy guns and toy helmets. He suggested that the mother take cover behind an armchair. He and the boy took cover behind another armchair. There was a shootout between the bad and the good guys. Then Ezra stood up and said, "OK, now is tomorrow and the good guys have already made peace with the bad guys."

The bugs that were busted in this intervention were horse blinders and flip-flop.

Eli's attitude toward his mother was inconsistent. When he was in a fit of rage, he would forget the loving relationship between his mother and himself. When the tantrum was over, he would forget how he had behaved and what he had said when he lost his self-control. The first play-therapeutic move was to turn the aggression into make-believe play. Eli could own his aggression and anger, but at the same time alienate himself from it. Eli's mother could, thanks to the basic duality of play, see the situation as it was – a war, but she also could, by virtue of the owning and alienation of play, understand that she had the right to defend herself.

The second play-therapeutic move, saying, "OK, now is tomorrow and the good guys have already made peace with the bad guys", was designed to bust Eli's flip-flop and horse blinders by owning and alienation. The idea was to bring to Eli's awareness, in the midst of the struggle, the temporariness of his tantrum and the unquestionable love between him and his mother. The expression "Now is tomorrow", which blends the future with the present, could have this effect.

Session 9.2 Daliah
After Daliah's family moved to another city for her father's work, she found it difficult to adapt to the new apartment and environment. Although the new environment was friendly, and she was well-received at the new school, she was unable to undergo a natural and proper adjustment process. For months she would continue to cry and demand to return to the previous apartment. The therapist, Emily, encouraged Daliah to create in the playroom, using play blocks, paintings, etc., an environment that represented her previous surroundings, her room, the view from her window, friends she had and more. Daliah and Emily played as if they were living in Daliah's former environment, before moving out. During the play Emily kept saying "Now is then" and "Here is there". Daliah enjoyed this play very much. It made it easier for her to adapt to the new place.

Later on, Emily helped Daliah create the opposite situation. She encouraged Daliah to create in the playroom an environment that represented her current surroundings. Then Emily and Daliah played as if the current environment, materialized as it were in the play room, was actually Daliah's previous life environment. Again, Emily used over and over again the expressions "Now is then" and "Here is there". Daliah liked this play too.

The main bug that was busted in this intervention was fifth wheel. Emily's proximity and attachment programs with respect to her previous life were no more relevant to the programs related to her new life. The bug busters that were used in this intervention were arbitrariness of a signifier (the raw materials of the playroom signified the previous environment) and owning and alienation (the old environment was realified. The raw materials of the play room were identicated with the old environment). However, the seriousness of the realification and identication were denied. Emily could enjoy "being in her previous life", while being aware of the reality of her current life situation. The owning the alienation operated in two opposite directions. In the first play, Daliah's previous life was realified as her current life. In the second play, her current life was realified as her previous life. The time and place of the play were identified with the time and place of her former life. In both cases there was also alienation. The two play sessions bridged between Daliah's previous life and her present life and de-emphasized the contrast between the two.

Another linguistic peculiarity of make-believe play is the frequent use of the past tense to directly indicate the realified time of the imaginary entity or event. Often this kind of past tense co-occurs with the use of the third person rather than the first- or second-person pronouns.

Suppose the following two sentences were said in the framework of make-believe play (rather than in the framework of storytelling). (a) "Let's pretend they were aliens" (instead of "Let's pretend we are aliens"); (b) "The wolf swallowed Granny". In both sentences the past tense ("were", "swallowed") does not indicate past time relative to the actual time of the play, but an imaginary time in which the players "are" aliens and the wolf "is swallowing" granny. One may say that in such sentences the actual time and place of the play are not identicated with the imagined time and place. The latter time and place are referred to directly. They are realified without being identicated. There is no "now" and "here", only "then" and "there". One can see a similarity between this use of the past tense in make-believe play and its use to indicate a hypothetical situation. An example of such use is the sentence, "Suppose the following two sentences *were* said in the framework of make-believe play."

In play therapy, the use of this type of past tense can serve as a way of distancing the realified content from the actual time and place of the play. In other words, this use of the past tense reinforces the player's alienation from the play content and weakens its owning.

Imagine a play therapy designed to serve as what has been termed *stress inoculation*. For example, a child is supposed to undergo an operation and a make-believe simulated operation is performed in the play room. Using this type of past tense and the third person is likely to reduce the child's level of fear from the procedure. "Let's pretend the doctor gave him an injection of anesthesia" would be less frightening than "Let's pretend the doctor is giving you an injection of anesthesia".

The verbal meta-cognition capacity of very young children is particularly evident in the ease with which they talk about their own play, plan it ahead, negotiate about it with their playmates, leave it to discuss it, comment on it and go back to it. Here are some examples:

Observation 9.1 Eric and Alina
Eric (6.8) and Alina (6.4) play in Eric's bedroom. Eric plays the role of a storyteller. He tells, feigning an affected voice of a narrator, a story about a brother and sister, Keeky and Kooka, who were often fighting. (Alina was not Eric's sister, she was his playmate). Then he and Alina start a rough-and-tumble mock fight, like two puppies. At some point the play becomes more violent. It turns out that Alina is stronger than Eric. She overcomes him and forces him to be lying on the bed. Eric is saying, "Stop it! It is not Keeky, it's the narrator!"

Eric found a clever way to save his face and stop Alina from having the upper hand. He stepped out of the make-believe role and spoke as himself, Eric, about this role. Alina wasn't supposed to fight with him if he was "the narrator" rather than Keeky.

Session 9.3 Ashley
Ashley (six) was always willing to only play roles in which she was the best in every way: The most athletic, the smartest and the most beautiful. In one of the sessions she played as if she was competing against imaginary professional acrobats in acrobatics exercises on a mattress. Indeed, she was good at simple tricks relative to her age. She demanded of her therapist Jo to make puppets representing her competitors trying to perform the same tricks, but to have them fail, fall and get hurt. At some point, she herself could not complete a trick and fell. She told Jo, "It's only make-believe, so let's pretend I didn't fall and did do the trick perfectly."

In another session, Ashley gave Jo the role of a prince, who was supposed to choose the most beautiful and smartest of three candidates for marriage with him. Two candidates were dolls and Ashley was the third candidate. To test the wisdom of the candidates, each of them had to solve three riddles. The two dolls were supposed to fail the quiz test, and Ashley (surprise!) was supposed to succeed. Jo made up three riddles. He made the two dolls give funny, stupid answers. Ashley didn't know the answers. She whispered to Jo, "Tell me the right answers, but in the play we'll make-believe that I did know the answers."

Obviously, Ashley's verbal moves attested to a clever though naive meta-cognition ability. She was aware of her own shortcomings and could clearly distinguish between these shortcomings in the real world and their imagined lack in the world of make-believe.

The following observation is copied from Ariel (2002, pp.80–82).

Observation 9.2 The power of good and the power of evil
Itamar and Ofer, both seven-years-old, were playing on the sofa in the living room of Itamar's home. Itamar occupied the right corner of the sofa and Ofer its left corner.

Itamar: Let's play Koory and Mari.
Ofer: Mari was the good one, like last time.
Itamar: I was Koory. Meefon, the commander of the bad ones, hypnotized me to kill Mari, even though he was my best friend.
   Itamar is wearing a fixed stare, like being hypnotized, stretching his two arms forward. His stare is directed at Ofer.
Ofer (declaring ceremonially): Evil, evaporate!
   He attaches the two palms of his hands to one another and then draws them apart abruptly.
   Itamar is walking slowly toward Ofer, his arms stretched forward, like a sleepwalker. Ofer stops him with the palms of his hands.

Ofer (speaking in a slow, authoritative voice): Your heart. You can control it. You can decide who you are.

    He stares directly into Itamar's eyes. Itamar bows slightly toward Ofer, and then raises his still stretched arms, standing motionless.

Ofer: Do something.

    Itamar turns his back on Ofer. He walks to the right corner of the sofa. He bends forward, bringing his face close to the sofa.

Itamar: I can see Meefon's face in the magic looking glass.

    He straightens up, turning the front of his body toward Ofer, stretching his arms forward again. He is looking at Offer like a sleepwalker.

Ofer: Are you again with the evil? That's clear. You were told you had the right to decide who you are, and you decided to be with the evil.

    Ofer takes an apron placed on a bench near the sofa, and continues speaking in a formal, monotonic voice.

Ofer: Sometimes one has to kill people in order to be good, and sometimes one has to imprison them, and that is the right thing to do. And that is (raising his voice) what I'm going to do.

    He ties Itamar's wrists with the apron. Itamar doesn't object.

Ofer: You won't be able to free yourself! Koory, for the sake of your friend Mari, who was trustful, will you decide who you are? A member of the powers of good or a member of the powers of evil?

    Itamar does not answer. He stretches his arms forward again, like a sleepwalker.

Itamar: My master!

Ofer: What do you mean?

Itamar: I am at your service. I was bad, but after I saw Meefon's face in the magic looking glass I understood my heart and became good.

Ofer: I don't want you to be at my service, I want you to be free and choose who you are.

Itamar: But if I am free, I'm afraid I'll be bad.

This seems to be a play Itamar and Ofer have not played for the first time, but they decided in advance about the division of roles. They clearly distinguished between play and non-play, as attested by their using play names. Their play moves certainly reflected a high level of meta-cognition. They used the make-believe as an arena for discussing philosophical questions such as free will, freedom of choice between good and evil and being controlled, under the spell of another being versus being liberated.

Summary of chapter 9

This chapter is devoted to a discussion of the linguistic peculiarities of make-believe play and their play-therapeutic applications. A frequently brought forward argument is challenged – that young children are incapable of activating verbal meta-cognition and therefore play is the preferable medium for child therapy. Meta-cognition is an inherent property of make-believe play. Children distinguish between play and non-play and often comment about the contents of their own play. One of the peculiar characteristics of the use of language in make-believe play is the ambiguity of expressions of time and place. Seemingly self-contradictory expressions, such as "Now is then" and "Here is there", refer to the time and place of playing ("now", "here") and to the imaginary make-believe time and place ("then" and "there"). Therefore, they are not self-contradictory. The use of such peculiar linguistic expressions in make-believe play has various advantages, which can be utilized in play therapy. Such expressions can serve as play bug-busters, because they invite the imaginary time and place to the real time and place of playing. Another linguistic peculiarity of make-believe play is the frequent use of the past tense to directly indicate the realified time of the imaginary entity or event. Often this kind of past tense co-occurs with the use of the third person, rather than the first- or second-person pronouns. In play therapy, the use of this type of past tense can serve as a way of distancing the realified content from the actual time and place of the play. In other words, this use of the past tense reinforces the player's alienation from the play content and weakens its owning.

The verbal meta-cognition capacity of very young children is particularly evident in the ease with which they talk about their own play, plan it ahead, negotiate about it with their playmates, go out of it to discuss it, comment on it and go back to it.

Assignments

Suggest play-therapeutic uses of the linguistic peculiarities of make-believe play (the ambiguity of expressions of time and place, the use of the past tense to indicate imaginary time and meta-play expressions discussing or commenting on the play content) as ways of busting bugs in Cases 1.1 (Rusella) and 3.2 (Kabr).

A classified list of publications

Play as a language

Ariel, S. (2002). *Children's imaginative play: A visit to Wonderland*. Westport, CT: Praeger.

Bruner, J. (1983). Play, thought and language. *Peabody Journal of Education* 60 (3).

Ely, R. and McCabe, A. (1994). The language play of kindergarten children. *First Language* 14 (40), pp.19–35.

Gandini, L. (2011). Play and the hundred languages of children: An interview with Lella Gandini. *American Journal of Play* 4 (1), pp.1–18.

Chapter 10

Make-believe play as a vehicle of learning and development

In Chapter 3, the internal and external subsystems are listed. Each of the subsystems and all of them can be looked at *synchronically* or *diachronically*. Both the external subsystems and the internal subsystems keep changing and developing. The diagnostic assessment and the therapy should take into account such changes and developments. It is also important to have a developmental profile of each client across all the internal systems that are relevant to the case.Development on all the developmental lines, in any of the internal subsystems, advances through the following dimensions: growth; internalization; complexity; coordination and integration; differentiation; depth of processing; concreteness vs. abstraction; flexibility; constancy and stability; objectivity; monitoring and control; socialization.

The difficulties brought to therapy may be described as manifestations of arrested development, on various developmental parameters, of programs belonging to any of the subsystems. There are mutual influences between developmental delays or regression on the one hand and the presence of bugs in the various programs. The bugs are energized by unbalanced emotions, and so are, in many cases, the developmental delays or regression. The therapy must restore the emotions to balance, so that the bugs can be eliminated, and the various programs can regain their ability to develop.

Children learn and develop while being engaged in play in general and make-believe play in particular. Play has this magic power. Play serves as a platform for learning and development in all dimensions, applying to any subsystem. If necessary, such learning and development can be assisted by play therapy. Learning and development-enhancing play-therapeutic moves can be administered to adults too.

Here are some examples:

Observation 10.1 Motor development – balance
A group of kindergarten children played as if they were storks standing on one leg. They made considerable efforts to maintain balance over time.

These efforts contributed to advancing the children's motor development on the dimensions of coordination and integration, flexibility, constancy and stability, monitoring and control.

Observation 10.2 Attention and perception
Sarah (5) and Rami (5.3) played with toy cars in the backyard of Rami's house. Sarah said, "But there are no roads here, only grass." The two kids began searching for something that could mark a road. Then Sarah had an idea: A black gardening hose could be used as a signifier for a road.

On another occasion, Sara and Rami played "family" in Sarah's home. Rami suggested "being Grandma sitting on a rocking chair and knitting." He was looking for knitting needles but couldn't find any. Then he found a silvery candy box with a lid attached to the body of the box by hinges. He began opening and closing the lid rhythmically, saying, "I'm knitting"

In both cases the children surveyed the environment, actively and purposefully directing their attention to potentially suitable objects. Their choice of objects was not obvious. Sarah abstracted the properties "black", "long" and perhaps "winding" from the hose and ignored the properties "flexibility" and "being narrow". Rami abstracted the property "movable in two directions" from the candy box and ignored all its other properties.

Such play activities promote learning and development of attention and visual perception on the dimensions of differentiation, depth of processing; concreteness vs. abstraction; flexibility and objectivity.

Observation 10.3 Creative thinking and problem-solving
Colin and Omar, both five years old, made a see-saw for dolls out of a board of wood placed on a can. The see-saw went off balance and fell. The boys didn't give up. They attempted to understand the causes for the failure and went on attempting to correct the errors and achieve equilibrium. In the course of their exchange they learned that they should find the center of gravity of the board in its midpoint and that the dolls should be of the same weight.

On another occasion they dug "a river" in the sand. Then they poured water into it from a pail, expecting the water to flow. It did not. They tried to find out why. After some discussion they realized the cause of the failure. The surface of the ground was flat rather than sloping.

In both cases the children discovered laws of physics on a practical level. Their play and the discussions around it were arenas for learning and development on the dimensions of depth of processing, concreteness vs. abstraction, objectivity and monitoring and control.

Observation 10.4 Memory, planning and organization
A group of five kindergarten children continued their regular space-travel play.

The group leader, Simon, said, "Today we are going to discover a new planet, Gravanar. Sean, today you must stay in the control tower because last week you were the spacecraft commander. Ella and Luna, you'll be the monstrous aliens inhabiting Gravanar."

Sean, Ella and Luna refused to play the undesirable roles assigned to them. Complex negotiations pursued. After the problems of roles has been resolved, the members of the group began planning the various aspects of the play, signifying objects. Locations, plot, etc.

This whole play activity and the discussions around it provided an opportunity for learning and development of many kinds, on all the developmental dimensions - memory, expanding the knowledge of the world, planning and organization, conflict resolution, postponement of gratification, social negotiations, pro-social behavior and more.

Observation 10.5 Self and body images and concepts

Eight-year-old Nico, a lanky, pale, weak, passive and shy boy was rejected and harassed by his peers who would call him "scarecrow". He told his 13-year-old sister Martha about his suffering. She had a maternal attitude toward him and was his sole playmate. In their make-believe play he was a scarecrow protecting the family's farm against birds of prey. Martha played the role of an eagle who gets scared when he sees the scarecrow. Then, like in *The Wizard of Oz*, the scarecrow came to life. He could speak and walk. Martha changed the rags he wore with superhero clothing. He could now fight birds of prey and predators with his own hands.

In this play, the bug-busters owning, and alienation and possible world were activated. Nico tried modes of behavior that were radically different from his usual patterns of behavior and internal experiences. The play could help him expand his repertoire of behaviors and internal experiences. His body and self-image could develop on the dimensions of growth, internalization, differentiation, depth of processing, flexibility, monitoring and control.

Observation 10.6 Self and body boundaries

Willow, aged four, was clinging to her eight-year-old sister, Joy. She would hug Joy, sit on her and imitate her movements, facial expressions and play activities. Joy found creative ways of drawing clear self and body boundaries between herself and Willow in make-believe play (proximity plans). One way was to give Willow creative and differentiated make-believe roles that also required keeping physical distance between herself and willow. For example, Joy suggested that her sister play the role of a whale living in the sea. She herself played the role of a mother who sailed with her little son (represented by a doll). The mother warned the boy who wanted to see the whale not to bend over the railing because he might fall into the water. The boy didn't listen to her and fell into the water. The whale caught him and saved him and returned him to his mother.

Willow enjoyed this play. It was reinforcing. It enabled her to experience having clear body and self-boundaries with Joy and still enjoying her attention, playing with her and being in an empowering and helpful role. The play with Joy helped willow learn and develop self and body boundaries on the dimensions of differentiation, flexibility, monitoring and control and socialization.

Observation 10.7 Empathy and pro-social attitude
Every conjoint play of children requires empathy and a pro-social attitude, otherwise it will fail. In addition, the play contents can reflect sensitivity and concern for others.

Children in a Kindergarten played with a toy puppy. They played as if he had been abandoned by his mother and was left alone, sick, hungry and miserable. They all participated in taking care of him. They brought him milk from a toy baby-bottle, covered him with a blanket, gave him food and hugged him.

The children experimented in being sensitive, empathetic and helpful. The play helped them develop on the dimensions of differentiation (differentiating between their own needs and wishes and the other person's), flexibility, objectivity (seeing the real needs of the other person) and socialization.

Observation 10.8 Self-control and postponing gratification
A group of children in a kindergarten played "a war between monsters and good magicians". When a monster caught a magician, the magician would become a monster, but if the magician managed to touch a monster with his finger before the monster could catch him, the monster would become a statue, unable to move.

The competition component in this game motivated the children to play by the rules. A monster that was paralyzed and unable to move was signified by a child who agreed and managed to control himself, to accept the fact that he had lost and to postpone his natural aggressive response. Such a game proves to impulsive children that they can control themselves if they want. It helps them develop on the dimensions of internalization (internalizing their impulses), flexibility, monitoring and control and socialization.

Interdisciplinary seminar

Shlomo: Let's see how the learning and development functions of make-believe play can be applied in play therapy. Consider the following case:

Case 10.1 Shan
Nine-year-old Shan was referred by his parents to Lace, a trainee of mine, a clinical psychologist and family therapist. The presenting complaint, as phrased by his mother Lara, was, "He thinks and behaves in black and white." His father, Nathan, added, "He has been like that since he was a baby, stubborn, rigid, unforgiving. He divides everything, the world, people, situations, us, into absolutely good or absolutely bad. We know of no one

he had learned this pattern from. He is our only child. We are very lenient, affordable and loving parents and reasonable people. It is his character. No other explanation."

Lara said, "If I say or do something he doesn't like, he can respond, 'I am not your son and you are not my mother. I'm going to leave home and never come back', and then he can ignore me and behave like I am a stranger, for days. Usually, he responds in this way to my well-meaning comments, such as that he should be cautious and not walk barefoot when the floor is wet, because he can fall and get hurt. I think he interprets what I say in a totally distorted way. Maybe he thinks I don't trust him, treat him like a baby who does not understand, or maybe he even thinks I want him to skid and fall and get hurt. But if someone, a friend or whoever, says a bad word about me, he protects me fiercely and says that I am the best mother in the world."

Nathan added, "He is like that with friends too, so they stay away from him and don't want his company."

Daniel: I want to understand the difference between low level of development and bugs that are energized by unbalanced emotions. I see in Shan's proximity-control plans, especially with respect to his mother and his friends, bugs like flip-flop – fluctuations between proximity and distance; non-sense – misinterpreting his mother's benevolent messages; and horse blinders – ignoring all data other than those relating to whether he is being mistreated.

Shlomo: True, but the question is whether these bugs are products of processes such as loss of simplicity, or reflections of a deep-seated low level of development in certain areas.

Ethan: If we look at it this way, I see a low level of cognitive development: a small repertoire, for his age, of concepts related to interpersonal relationships (relevant dimension – growth); simplistic conceptualizations (relevant dimensions – complexity; coordination and integration; differentiation; depth of processing; concreteness vs. abstraction); misjudgment of social messages (relevant dimension – objectivity); inability to keep a consistent image or concept of another person (relevant dimension – constancy, stability and socialization); low level of internalization of social norms (relevant dimensions – internalization, socialization)

Lailah: These are not just cognitive programs. I see a low level of differentiation of emotional nuances; under-development of internalization of caretakers; no consistent attachment; egocentricity and narcissism more than empathy and pro-social attitude; and low reality testing.

Anna: Is he on the autistic spectrum, Asperger's perhaps?

Shlomo: I prefer not to tag him. Our purpose is to explore ways of using play therapy to enhance his development on the various subsystems and dimensions you mentioned.

Ethan: I have an idea how to use play to help Shan develop a better ability to internalize and keep a constant image of caretakers, especially his mother, and acquire consistent attachment. There are many videos on YouTube that show how you can merge different pictures into one picture, using photoshop or other photo-editing software. It is easy to blend and merge two images of the same person into one image. I'd show Shan such videos. Then, in the make-believe role of a computer technician, I would "install a photoshop software in his brain". Next, we'd look together at various pictures of Shan's mother in a family pictures album. I'll ask Shan to close his eyes and merge his mother's various pictures into one picture, using the photoshop program I had installed in his brain. Later, we would re-create, in make-believe play, situations in which he was angry at his mother. I'd sit next to a computer mouse and keyboard and tell him that every time he gets angry at his mother, I'll turn on the image-blending program in his brain. The program will merge his mother's figures in all kinds of situations into a single figure. I'd give him a remote-control device and suggest that when he is angry at his mother, he himself will turn on the image-blending program in his brain.

Anna: Ingenious!

Shlomo: I agree, very original and creative. How would you explain the therapeutic effect of this intervention?

Daniel: Internalized objects keeps developing on the dimensions of complexity, coordination and integration, depth of processing, constancy and stability across variations of situational contexts, time and place. The play that Ethan invented can assist, using suggestion, these developmental processes, by instilling in Shan's mind a more constant, stable and integrated image of Shan's mother, irrespective of his momentary feelings. This play intervention could help Shan monitor and control this process.

Lailah: I would like to propose a play therapy intervention to help Shan develop basic trust and an ability to interpret and judge social messages correctly.

I would suggest to Shan that we both participate in a puppet show. His puppet will be "the boy". He will choose a name for the boy. My puppet will be "the boy's guardian angel". The role of the guardian angel will be to take care of the boy and get him out of trouble. The boy will not trust the guardian angel, will believe that he only pretends to be well-meaning, that he really is a malevolent hypocrite.

We'll play a scene in which the guardian angel tries to help the boy, gives him advice and warns him of dangers. The boy will not believe him, will be angry with him and sever all contacts with him.

Afterward I will start an argument between two dolls, a distrustful doll and a trusting doll. The distrustful doll will argue that the boy is right, that the guardian angel is only pretending to be good. The trusting doll will claim that the boy is wrong, the guardian angel has only good intentions. The trusting doll will suggest, "Let's ask the boy why he doesn't trust the guardian angel." The distrustful doll will agree. It is highly likely that Shan would refuse to answer. The trustful doll will say, "I know what to do. I have a device that reads minds. I'll turn it on and see who's right." I'll turn on the device to read the boy's thoughts. I will make noises and say that it is hard to hear the child's thoughts because of background noise. I'll make an effort to listen and say out loud things I've heard, without being sure I've heard them correctly.

I expect that it will be possible to see from Shan's mainly non-verbal reactions whether I hit the target or not. Then the instrument will be activated again, and I will utter the thoughts of the guardian angel, expressing concern for the boy, and sorrow that the boy doesn't allow the guardian angel to help and protect him.

Shlomo: Nice. How would this play therapy intervention help Shan develop an ability to interpret and judge social messages correctly?

Ethan: The basic duality of play is supposed to bring to Shan's awareness that he suspects the intentions of those who care for him and perhaps misinterprets these intentions. The play can allow him to "hear" the inner thoughts of the guardian angel and of himself and therefore perhaps doubt his negative interpretation. This play is designed to bust the bugs horse blinders and non-sense in his mind.

Daniel: These bugs are deep seated in his mind. Therefore, they reflect a low level of development of social communication.

Shlomo: You invented good examples. In later sessions we'll see how the use of play as a tool for learning and development is applied in more complete descriptions of cases.

Summary of chapter 10

Children learn and develop while being engaged in play in general and make-believe play in particular. Play serves as a platform for learning and development in all dimensions, applying to any subsystem. If necessary, such learning and development can be assisted by play therapy. Learning and development-enhancing play-therapeutic moves can be administered to adults too. Examples are given of the contribution of natural play to learning and development in the cognitive and psychomotor subsystems and in the personality development subsystems, on various developmental dimensions. Play-therapeutic applications of the power of play to promote learning and development are illustrated and discussed.

Assignments

1. Invent examples of play-therapeutic moves that apply the power of make-believe play as a promoter of learning and development in cognitive and psychomotor programs (e.g. perception, memory, language, conceptualization, creative thinking and problem-solving, motor aptitude). Analyze your examples in terms of the developmental dimensions (growth, internalization, complexity, etc.).

2. Same as 1, with respect to personality development programs (e.g. self and body images and concepts, self and body boundaries, attachment, egocentricity and narcissism vs. empathy and prosocial attitude, reality testing and self-control).

A classified list of publications

Play as a promoter of learning and development

Ariel, S. (2002). *Children's imaginative play: A visit to Wonderland* Westport, CT: Praeger.
Ariel, S. (2018). *Multi-dimensional therapy with families, children and adults: The Diamond Model.* London, UK: Routledge.
Frost, J.L., Wortham, S.C. and Reifel, S.C. (2011). *Play and child development.* London, UK: Pearson.
Singer, D., Michnik Golkoff, R. and Hirsch-Pasek, K. (2009). *Play = learning: How play motivates and enhances children's cognitive and social-emotional growth.* Oxford, UK: Oxford University Press.

Child learning and development through play therapy

Bratton, S., Ray, D. and Rhine, T. (2005). The efficacy of play therapy with children: A meta-analytic review of treatment outcomes. *Professional Psychology: Research and Practice* 36 (4), pp.376–390.
Schaefer, Ch.E. and Drewes, A. (2013). *The therapeutic powers of play: 20 core agents of change.* Hoboken, NJ: John Wiley and Sons.

Chapter 11

Make-believe play as a pacifier

The emotion-balancing mechanism of make-believe play is one instance of a much wider mechanism governing the dynamic interactions between emotions and cognitions.

In a person's spontaneous mental life there is no such entity as pure thoughts or pure emotions. What do exist are complex networks of associations between thoughts, feelings, sensations and emotions. These networks are organized around the person's *emotives*. An emotive is a theme with which a person is deeply preoccupied throughout her life or in a particular period of her life, a theme that arouses in her powerful emotions. For example, a person is troubled throughout her life with the thought that her mother has never loved her. This thought, whether well-founded or not, arouses in her powerful emotions of sadness, self-pity and anger. Another person is preoccupied in a particular period of his life with thoughts about his state of health. These thoughts are accompanied by acute anxiety.

Many emotives are not exclusive to a specific person but shared by many people of the same age or the same cultural background. The emotive "fear of being physically injured" is very common in children, mainly boys, of kindergarten and early school age, because at this age many children feel independent, strong, energetic, curious and adventurous on the one hand, and on the other are still very aware of their own vulnerability. The emotive "guilt feelings associated with failure to observe religious commandments" is prevalent among orthodox Jews. There are universal emotives, common to all or most human beings, such as fear of death.

The emotionally loaded theme of an emotive (e.g. "doubt with respect to mother's love") is only a general title designating an enormous, potentially infinite, field of private associations that are tied in the subjective mind of a specific person with the theme in question. Consider for instance the emotive "doubt with respect to mother's love". A person whose emotive it is will respond with arousal of sadness, self-pity and rage whenever relevant childhood or adult memories emerge in her mind. Obviously, memories interpreted as direct manifestations of rejection on the side of the mother are relevant, but not all relevant stimuli are such direct manifestations. The same person can have a similar, though not so intense, emotional response, for instance, after having seen a cat weaning her kittens by exposing her teeth and claws at them when they approach her udders. This person will be flooded with similar emotions when overhearing the song "Sometimes I feel like a motherless child". She will experience similar, though somewhat weaker emotions after having heard her son complain that his teacher ignores him.

To sum up, some of the relevant stimuli are closer to the thematic focal point, or nucleus, of an emotive. These are likely to arouse more powerful emotions. Other relevant stimuli are farther removed from this focal point. They are closer to the margins or periphery of the emotive's association network. The latter will arouse weaker emotions. It should be stressed that not only emotive-relevant thematic materials retrieved from memory arouse powerful emotions. Our brain seems to give priority to processing materials associated with our emotives. All the higher mental functions – attention, visual, auditory, olfactory and tactile sensory reception and perception, memory, creative and associative thought processes and motivation for action, etc., are sensitized to our emotives. Take for instance a person whose emotive is fear of being involved in a road accident. On the road, his attention, sensory sensitivity, visual, auditory, and even olfactory perception will be alerted to stimuli associated with this emotive, more than with stimuli that are not associated with this emotive. He will pay special attention to stimuli such as traffic lights, screeching of breaks and cars that travel too fast and do not keep distance from other cars. He will be highly sensitive to the smell of gasoline. He will recall accidents in which he was involved or which he witnessed.

Creative imagination is sensitized to emotives too. In a test, a man was asked to invent a free combination of two images. He came up with the combination "a bottle gun", and immediately realized that this was related to his childhood memory of his father terrorizing the family when drunk. Artists and authors very often create works that are inspired by their emotives. Likewise, motivation for action is influenced by one's emotives. A person whose emotive is fear of a road accident will take more precautions than a person who does not have such an emotive. For example, he will install special safety devices in his car and will drive more slowly and carefully.

Input stimuli and memory materials that are closer to the focal point, the nucleus of an emotive's associative field, have priority with respect to the right of access into all the processing channels. If, however, focal materials of an emotive arouse unbearable emotions, these materials lose their priority of access in favor of more peripheral materials. This process seems to be partly equivalent to the activation of the defense mechanism of displacement.

There are also extreme cases, in which the emotive materials are so troubling, that they are totally erased from one's conscious mind. Defense mechanisms such as repression and denial seem to be such cases.

The cognitive-affective mechanism described above may be seen as a cybernetic mechanism, a homeostatic feedback system that regulates and balances the intensity of emotional arousal brought about by the contents associated with the emotives. The emotive-related input, or the materials retrieved from memory, fan the emotional flames. If the flames reach an unbearable peak, the cybernetic feedback mechanism lowers the flames to a tolerable level by various means discussed below. The temporary calm achieved in this way again leads to an increase in the level of the flames, sometimes to an intolerable level, and the cycle repeats itself. This cycle serves as an emotion-balancing mechanism.

The emotion-balancing mechanism of make-believe play is one specific instance or subset of this general cybernetic mechanism. The signified, realified contents of the play are taken from the player's memory materials and their creative combinations. The selection of non-verbal identicated signifiers requires allocation of attention, using the senses and activating one's perception. Therefore, all the above hypotheses apply to the choice of play signifiers and signified contents straightforwardly. Mental contents that belong to the association fields of the player's emotives are more likely to be realified in his or her play than mental contents that do not belong to these association fields. Mental contents that are closer to the core (focal point, nucleus) of an emotive's field of associations will have easier access to the player's make-believe play than mental contents that belong to the periphery of this field. However, if the choice and realification of core contents cause an intolerable level of emotional arousal, the player will replace the core contents with peripheral contents or will introduce into his play other emotion-balancing techniques, to be discussed below, until he or she calms down and is ready to raise the level of emotional arousal again, and the cycle repeats itself. The same applies to the signifiers, the entities identicated with the realified contents. Tangible entities that seem to be related to the player's emotive, especially if they seem to be associated with the core of the emotive, are more likely to draw the player's attention, to be sensed and perceived as relevant to the realified content. Therefore, they are more likely to be identicated with the realified contents. But if these entities contribute to arousing the emotions beyond a tolerable peak, they are likely to be replaced by other tangible entities which are less arousing.

Session 11.1 Rex
Eight-year-old Rex participated in a group play therapy. He was a strong, athletic boy who assumed leadership in the group. One day he lay on the carpet, pretending to be ill. One of the girls in the group took the role of a doctor. She tested him, using a toy stethoscope. He closed his eyes and lay flat-legged, as if he had passed out. Then he got up and said, "I am dead," and walked limply with his eyes closed to the pile of pillows in the corner of the room. He lay down and covered himself with large cushions. He whispered, "I'm dead, I'm buried," and fell silent. I put on a hat that could pass for a doctor's cap and told the girl who played the doctor, "I'm the ward manager. I think he is still alive. We'll take him out and give him resuscitation."

Rex whispered, "No, I'm completely dead. I'm buried very deep and no one can get me out of the grave." He covered himself with more and more pillows. I asked the girl doctor and the rest of the group, "What can we do?

Do you have any suggestions?" Suddenly Rex jumped up and out from under the pile of pillows, clearly in panic. He ran around the room shouting, "I'm a ghost! I'm a ghost! No air here! There is no air!" Then he took a ball, sat down on a chair and said, "Ghosts can play football too."

This was a very uncharacteristic play of Rex. I asked his mother if anyone has fallen ill or died in the family. She said, "Yes, his father got leukemia, but Rex doesn't know it." I told her, "I have news for you, he does know it."

One can see clearly the cybernetic mechanism of emotional balance in this example. Since Rex learned of his father's illness, he developed an emotive "fear of disease and death", not only of his father but also of himself. He realified the mental images of illness and death and identicated himself, his body postures, the pillows etc., with these images. He stepped up and escalated the illness and death expressions, culminating in being buried deep, irreversibly, in his grave. This was an expression of the peak, the hard nucleus of his emotive. At that point the fear arousal was intolerable, reaching a level of panic, so he gradually de-escalated the play, going to images that belong to the periphery of the emotive, such as going out of the grave as a ghost, and then returning, "as a ghost", to his favorite ball play.

The CDCA technique introduced in Chapter 6 displays this emotional balancing mechanism.

Interdisciplinary seminar

Lailah: You mentioned that children in their play employ all kinds of emotion-balancing techniques. You said some of these techniques resemble defense mechanisms like repression and displacement.

Shlomo: That's right. I have learned emotion-balancing techniques children use from many years of observing children playing. Some kids are really, really good at it. Here is a list of such techniques. I suppose it is a partial list, not covering all the ingenious emotion- balancing techniques children use in their make-believe play.

Repetition in a safe environment

When emotive-related themes are repeated over and over again in the safe environment of play, a habituating, positively reinforcing effect is created. The player, as the director of the play and as an actor, experiences a sense of mastery over the emotionally unbalanced themes and events that are realified in his or her play.

Lailah: I see it in Rusella's play. In the session I reported about (Session 1.1), there was a part in which she made the doll that apparently represented herself sleep in the forest, and then monkeys came and threw her into a wastepaper basket. At that point she became a ghost. She repeated this scene in each of the following sessions.

Daniel: Like Rex in Shlomo's example, she became a ghost.

Lailah: I was asking myself why she did keep repeating a scene in which she was treated terribly, thrown into the trash, left to die.

Shlomo: Sigmund Freud tried to contend with this question in his article *Beyond the Pleasure Principle* (2011), referring to repeated dreams of traumatized soldiers of the First Word War, as well as to a child's play. He came up with answers that reflect what in current terminology are termed *habituation, positive reinforcement* and *mastery*, although he didn't use the same words. Habituation – when you repeat the same bad experience over and over again it takes the sting out of the initial powerful experience. Positive reinforcement – the difficult experience is played repeatedly in the safe and pleasant environment of the play. The denial of seriousness strengthens the sense of safety. Mastery – the player is not a passive, helpless victim. He or she is the one who decides to realify these themes and can initiate and stop it at will. The player, as the director of the play, can also look at the experience, as it were, from aside or above, and inspect it objectively (basic duality), figuring out what it is about. Since Freud, all the main methods for treating anxiety and trauma have been based on these principles.

Ups and downs (fluctuations)

This mechanism has been discussed above. As in the case of Rex, the player is moving from play behaviors reflecting unbalanced emotions to behaviors reflecting balanced emotions and then back to unbalanced emotions. This is especially noticeable when the emotional imbalance reaches the hard core or nucleus of the emotive and becomes unbearable. The cycle repeats itself.

Distancing

Signified contents and signifiers belonging to the core of the player's emotives can be replaced by themes and signifiers belonging to the emotives' periphery, until the player is ready to introduce core themes and signifiers again.

Observation 11.1 Lee
In a make-believe play, Lee, whose emotive was a fear of being drowned (related to an event in which he almost drowned), used to bring into his play the theme of a submarine that loses its oxygen generator and cannot emerge to the sea surface. He changed "submarine" into a "boatsy submarine", which is a boat whose lower, submerged part, is a submarine. Later he turned the boatsy submarine into just a boat. The submarine that lost its oxygen generator belonged to the hard core of his emotive. The boatsy submarine was more marginal, closer to the periphery, and the ordinary boat was yet closer to the periphery.

Anna: The idea of a boatsy submarine is so cute!
Shlomo: Often childlike combinations of this kind belong to a transitional stage between the center, core of the emotive and more marginal parts of the emotive's associative field, or between an area in the periphery and an area that is more distant from the core of the emotive.
Lailah: You said that distancing is like displacement as a defense mechanism?
Shlomo: Not exactly the same, similar. Displacement is the redirecting of thoughts, feelings and impulses directed at one person or object, but taken out upon another person or object. Displacement can also be the transferring of a strong emotion from the original object to another object, for instance to a diver instead of a submarine. But, unlike in displacement, distancing often involves transformation. The original theme that is closer to the core of the emotive is transformed into something else, more far-removed from the core, e.g. Rex in Session 11.1 transformed himself into a ghost. As a ghost he was still "dead" but wasn't buried and could move freely in the open air.

Introducing protective devices or curing agents

Often, when children introduce into their play dangerous, scary contents, they balance the aroused fear by introducing into their play people or objects who protect or cure the threatened or injured figure in the play. Lee (Observation 11.1), who introduced the theme of "drowning submarines" into his play, took a toy doctor's toolbox and called it "a red-cross submarine". In Observation 6.2 Tamar played as if the baby princess ate soap and was sick. She was cured when her mother breastfed her.

Empowering and immunization

This is similar to introducing protective devices or curing agents. The difference is that in empowering and immunization the player doesn't introduce into his play a figure or device external to the protagonist but reinforces or immunizes the protagonist himself. For example, a boy who was afraid of being a victim of violence, played as if his skin was turned into a steel shield.

Neutralizing

The child neutralizes the dangerous or threatening object or figure by weakening it, depriving it of its power.

Observation 11.2 Rana

Five-year-old Rana, who played with a threatening toy shark in a children's group therapy, told her playmate Bob (as if from the mouth of the shark), "Don't worry, I'm hollow." Bob feared the shark and was unable to relax. The therapist played as if she were a dentist who came to treat the shark because "he has weak teeth".

Compensation

The player compensates herself in play for deprivation or deficiency.

A girl from a poor family played as if she was a princess living in a palace, wearing the most expensive, beautiful clothes and eating the best food and sweets.

Reversing

Turning weakness into strength

Observation 11.3 John and Leo
Five-year-old John and Leo, who were friends and neighbors, used to be harassed by a boy named Eric in their Kindergarten. At home they would take a rather violent revenge on a doll they named Eric.

Observation 11.4 Paul
Nine-year-old Paul, who suffers from muscle weakness (hypotonia), played games that expressed his weakness. The therapist gave him a light black plastic sports weights and played with him as if he were a professional weight-lifter.

Stopping

Observation 11.5 Ian
Ian, who was angry at his mother, threw a woman doll from a window sill. He said he threw her from the roof of a building into the streets. He caught the doll before it reached the floor and said the woman was stopped in the air by an invisible balloon.

Ethan: Do kids who play really feel all these emotions? From my experience, children who play with the most horrible things are calm and enjoying themselves, as if they do not feel these things at all. Do they employ defense mechanisms such as denial and repression?

Shlomo: It varies from child to child. There are children whose play does put them into intolerable emotional pressures, especially traumatized children. They can be re-traumatized by their play. But I am not sure that the relative calmness of children who bring to their play difficult contents stems from the use of defense mechanisms such as repression, denial or emotional isolation. It seems that the calm results mainly from the essence of make-believe play, from the fact that the child creates an imaginary world, that he knows it's just play. It's like we enjoy horror movies because we know it's only a movie. Still, some adults are terrified by horror movies. They don't succeed in isolating themselves from the horror, because the movie touches their central emotives.

Daniel: But you yourself alluded to defense mechanisms. I somehow feel that the emotional balancing techniques you listed are related to defense mechanisms, but I'm not sure I can say exactly how.

Shlomo: I would say that make-believe play in general and in particular the emotion-balancing techniques employed by players are related and not related to defense mechanisms. The main difference, as I see it, is that defense mechanisms are unconscious and uncontrolled whereas the emotion-regulation functions of make-believe play have defensive power; like defense mechanisms, they are conscious and controlled. In make-believe play, the player chooses which contents to bring to the play and how to express them, and yet does not take them seriously and does not believe they represent something real.

I must add a reservation. The concepts of defense mechanisms are very complex and multi-faceted. They have different interpretations in different theoretical frameworks.

Here is a case in which the emotion-balancing mechanisms of play didn't work:

Case 11.1 Bella
Eight-year-old Bella was sexually abused by an uncle. Every time this event was mentioned, Bella would have an unbearable stomach ache and start crying and shouting. She refused to talk about this traumatic experience.

In play therapy sessions Bella was reproducing the violation without censorship. She would take off her panties and make a man doll touch her. Then she would go into a whirl, crying that she had a stomach ache. The play failed to sooth her. It re-traumatized her. Later she would do the same with dolls, without involving her own body. But she would panic again. The emotion-balancing techniques of play were not available to her. Her play was too literal. The repetition did not have the habituating effect.

Try to think of ideas for being accepted to the play and help her use some of the techniques discussed above.

Ethan: I would start with relaxation techniques. Then I would frame the situation as a joint make-believe play. Maybe I'd suggest that we do a puppet theater or a movie. I would make non-human puppets available, such as the wolf and Little Red Riding Hood or even less obvious choices, such as a cat lying in wait for a mouse, a pickpocket or the like. This already would be an application of distancing, because it would take Bella's play away from the core of her emotive to slightly more peripheral parts. I could also suggest that the play happened on a make-believe planet or in Wonderland. I would turn myself into a welcoming alien or some other non-threatening creature, like a funny but wise clown or an owl.

Anna: I would start with introducing a protective device or figure, e.g. a watchdog.

Daniel: We could use empowering and immunization, like turning her skin into a shield, or reversing – making her big and the perpetrator small.
Lailah: Neutralizing – turning the bad one into a statue, paralyzed. Reversing – going into a time machine that takes her back to the time before she was abused.
Anna: I would use compensations such as prosecuting the figure representing the attacker, punishing him, restricting him.
Lailah: We can use ups and downs, help her fluctuate between images closer to the core of her emotive and images closer to its periphery.
Shlomo: The play-therapeutic uses of these emotion-balancing techniques are controlled applications of natural emotion-balancing uses of play, observed in children's spontaneous play activities. The main play-therapeutic effect of these techniques is preparing the ground for the operation of other play bug-busters. Since bugs are energized by unbalanced emotional responses to stress, clients are more likely to be receptive to corrective information after their relevant emotion-balance has at least partly been restored.

Summary of chapter 11

The emotion-balancing mechanism of make-believe play is one instance of a much wider mechanism governing the dynamic interactions between emotions and cognitions. These dynamic interactions revolve around the person's *emotives*. An emotive is a theme with which a person is deeply preoccupied throughout her life or in a particular period of her life, a theme that arouses in her powerful emotions. Every such theme constitutes a complex, potentially endless, network of associations between thoughts, feelings, sensations and emotions. Many emotives are not exclusive to a specific person but are shared by many people of the same age or the same cultural background. Some of the associations are closer to the thematic focal point, or nucleus, of an emotive. These are likely to arouse more powerful emotions. Other relevant stimuli are further removed from this focal point. They are closer to the margins or periphery of the emotive's association network. The latter will arouse weaker emotions. Our brain gives priority to processing materials associated with our emotives. All the higher mental functions – attention, visual, auditory, olfactory and tactile sensory reception and perception, memory, creative and associative thought processes and motivation for action are sensitized to our emotives. Input stimuli and memory materials that are closer to the focal point or the nucleus of an emotive's associative field have priority with respect to the right of access into all the processing channels. If, however focal materials of an emotive arouse unbearable emotions, these materials lose their priority of access in favor of more peripheral materials. This cognitive-affective mechanism is a cybernetic mechanism, a homeostatic feedback system that regulates and balances the intensity of emotional arousal brought about by the contents associated with the emotives. The emotive-related input, or the materials retrieved from memory, fan the emotional flames. If the flames reach an unbearable peak, the cybernetic feedback mechanism lowers the flames to a tolerable level by various means. The temporary calm achieved in this way again leads to an increase in the level of the flames, sometimes to an intolerable level, and the cycle repeats itself. This cycle serves as an emotion-balancing mechanism. All the above hypotheses apply to the choice of play signifiers and signified contents straightforwardly. Mental contents that belong to the association fields of the player's emotives are more likely to be realified in his or her play than mental contents that do not belong to these association fields. Mental contents that are closer to the core of an emotive's field of associations will have easier access to the player's make-believe play than mental contents that belong to the periphery of this field. However, if the choice and realification of core contents arouse an intolerable level of emotional arousal, the player will replace the core contents with peripheral contents, or will introduce other emotion-balancing techniques, until he or she calms down and is ready to raise the level of emotional arousal again and the cycle repeats itself. The same applies to the signifiers, the entities identicated with the realified contents. Tangible entities that seem to be related to the player's emotives, especially if they seem to be associated with the core of the emotive, are more likely to draw the player's attention, to be sensed and perceived as relevant to the realified content. Therefore, they are more likely to be identicated with the realified contents. But if these entities contribute to arousing the emotions beyond a tolerable peak, they are likely to be replaced by other tangible entities, less arousing. Children use various emotion-balancing techniques in their make-believe play. These techniques are governed by the cybernetic mechanism described above. If a player is not adept at using such techniques, she can be assisted by a play therapist who teaches her such techniques or helps her applying them. Such techniques are listed, explained and illustrated. The list includes *repetition in a safe environment, ups and downs (fluctuations), distancing, introducing protective devices or curing agents, empowering and immunization, neutralizing, compensation, reversing* and *stopping*. The question is discussed whether children really feel powerful emotions when they play. The emotion-balancing techniques are related to but not identical with defense mechanisms. The similarities and differences between the former and the latter are discussed. Play-therapeutic applications of make-believe play emotion-balancing are considered.

Assignments

1. In the cases described below, the clients are in a state of emotional imbalance. For each example, suggest emotion-balancing moves of the following kinds: repetition in a safe environment, ups and downs (fluctuations), distancing, introducing protective devices or curing agents, empowering and immunization, neutralizing, compensation, reversing and stopping. If you think of other types of emotional balancing moves, please suggest them too. Analyze the emotional balancing mechanism in each example.

> **Case 11.2 Erez**
> Nine-year-old Erez, the son of a depressed single mother, was a strong, well-built boy, who at home behaved like an angel, to protect his mother against any further difficulty. At school he was harassed, attacked and ridiculed by the boys because of his being "a sissy". In a play therapy session, he understood that he was allowed to express himself freely and would have no censorship on any imaginative content he might project into the toys. He then began to take symbolic revenge on his schoolmates and on his absent father by '"killing", "torturing", "burying" and "mutilating" little dolls representing boys and a man. His whole play behavior was extremely aggressive. He was over-excited. But immediately after the session his mother called and said he had such an acute anxiety attack that she had to take him to emergency. The therapist understood that the play in the session broke his defenses. A therapeutic error was committed. Since Erez had not introduced emotion-balancing devices into his play, the therapist had to help him introduce such devices.
>
> **Case 11.3 Meera**
> (b) Eleven-year-old Meera lost her only true friend, a classmate, Rena, when the latter left the country with her parents. Meera exhibited unbalanced mourning reactions for months. She would cry incessantly and refuse to have any contact with any of her schoolmates.

A classified list of publications

Theories of emotions

Ekman, P., Friesen, W.V. and Ellsworth, Ph. (1972). *Emotions in the human face.* Amsterdam, The Netherlands: Elsevier.

Izard, C.E. (1977). *Human emotions.* New York, NY: Plenum Press.

Rogers, S. (2013). *The polyvagal theory: Neurophysiological foundations of emotions, attachment, communication and self-regulation.* New York, NY: W.W. Norton.

Tomkins, S.S. (1991). *Affect, imagery, consciousness: The negative affects: Anger and fear.* New York, NY: Springer.

Emotion-balancing functions of make-believe play

Ariel, S. (2002). *Children's imaginative play: A visit to Wonderland.* Westport, CT: Praeger.

Campbell, M.M and Knoetze, J.J. (2010). Repetitive symbolic play as a therapeutic process in child-centered play therapy. *International Journal of Play Therapy* 19 (4), pp.222–234.

Freud, S. (2011). *Beyond the pleasure principle.* Critical edition. Peterborough, ON, Canada: Broadview Press.

Phillips, R. (1994). A developmental perspective on emotions in play therapy. *International Journal of play therapy* 3 (2), pp.1–19.
Piaget, J. (2013). *Play, dreams and imitation in childhood.* London, UK: Routledge.

Defense mechanisms

Freud, A. (1992). *The ego and mechanisms of defence.* London, UK: Routledge.
Goody, J. (2017). *Defense mechanisms.* Houston, TX: Phosphene Publishing.

Chapter 12

The therapeutic powers of play, revisited

The attempts to describe and explain the therapeutic powers of play have had a considerable impact on the field. Schaefer and Drewes (2014) list the following major therapeutic powers of play: (a) Facilitating communication (self-expression, access to the unconscious, direct teaching, indirect teaching); (b) Fostering emotional wellness (catharsis, abreaction, positive emotions, counter-conditioning of fears, stress inoculation, stress management); (c) Enhancing social relationships (therapeutic relationship, attachment, social competence, empathy); and (d) Increasing personal strength (creative problem solving, resiliency, moral development, accelerated psychological development, self- regulation, self-esteem).

The contribution of this attempt to describe and corroborate the therapeutic powers of play to the development of the field of play therapy cannot be overestimated. It constitutes a much needed effort to integrate play theory and research with the applied art of play therapy. The hypotheses concerning the therapeutic powers of play are backed up by a huge amount of research evidence.

In this chapter, this contribution will be re-examined with a view to make some suggestions at improvements. The following discussion will take into consideration the examination of the nature of play, notably make-believe play in some of the previous chapters.

Crucial distinctions

In order to evaluate the validity of the various hypotheses concerning the therapeutic powers of play, it is not enough to look at play as a single monolithic entity, which is seen as an independent variable, with play-therapeutic procedures and processes as dependent variables. Clear, rigorous, formal definitions and distinctions, which can be operationalized, are required, in order to distinguish between play and non-play, between different kinds of play and between specific curative properties of each kind of play. Such definitions and distinctions are proposed in Chapters 8 and 9.

It is also needed to distinguish between therapeutic powers of play and therapeutic and didactic powers of play therapy.

I shall now briefly examine each of the categories of therapeutic powers of play described by the various contributors to Schaefer and Drewes (2014).

Facilitating communication

Self-expression

Some kinds of play are definitely media of self-expression, but so are numerous other forms of behavior – speech, shouts, crying, singing, body language, art, music, storytelling and so on. The challenge is to pinpoint and define those aspects of self-expression in play that have specific curative powers. As before, I'll focus on make-believe play. The concept of make-believe play is formally defined in Chapter 8. Its linguistic peculiarities and its various functions are discussed in Chapters 8–11.

The differential play-therapeutic advantages of verbal and non-verbal self-expression in make-believe play, as opposed to other forms of self-expression, are derived from its special nature, its simultaneous activation of verbal or non-verbal realification, identication and denial of seriousness. The play bug-busters of basic duality, owning and alienation, arbitrariness of the signifier and possible worlds are deduced from this very definition. These bug-busters make it easier for the player to bypass censorship, to express thoughts and feelings that belong to the core or periphery of her emotives (see Chapter 11), but are considered inappropriate, forbidden or shameful. For example, a girl whose emotive is fear that her mother does not want her can depict her in her play as a witch who is poisoning a baby girl. These play bug-busters also give the player legitimacy to express and explore ideas that are usually perceived as absurd, strange, unrelated to reality, but still belong to the field of associations of the player's emotives. For example, a boy can play as if he is an alien the size of the earth, who extinguishes the sun, causing the annihilation of every living creature. Thanks to the basic duality of make-believe play, the player can examine different parts of his own personality and various potential situations, while he is both an insider and an outsider, watching them in real time and place as an objective observer, as it were. A six-year-old girl can play as if she is a toddler and then as if she is an adult. From the standpoint of her real age, she is looking at what it is like to be a baby and what it is like to be an adult.

Access to the unconscious

Some of the founding parents of play therapy, such as Melanie Klein (1975), have argued that children's play is like free associations and dreams in adults, which are supposed to serve as entries to the unconscious. True, the make-believe play of preschoolers is often associative, but so is their spontaneous speech and the stories they make up. It is not the make-believe play that is associative but its realified contents.

There are considerable differences between make-believe play and dreams. In dreams there is no denial of seriousness. There is no distinction between the time and place of the dreaming and the time and place of the dreamt materials. The dreamer cannot choose or deliberately create the contents and structure of the dream. The dreamer can see people, objects and places he has never seen in his waking life and hear voices and sounds he has never heard in his waking life. True, in make-believe play the player can also realify imagined people, creatures and situations, but she does not see or hear vivid, hallucination-like visual and auditory images. In dreams, such images keep transforming into other images. Such transformations occur in make-believe play too. For example, in Tamar's play (Observation 6.1) she turned a realified image of herself as "a huge and beautiful girl", identicated by coquettish, graceful movements, into a realified image of herself as "a huge, scary dragon", identicated by a toy dragon. And then she said that this was just a disguise. In make-believe play, however, such transformations are created deliberately as a part of the play's emotion-balancing mechanism, whereas in dreams they are an inherent structural feature.

Perhaps instead of talking about access to the unconscious, it would be more accurate to say that verbalized realification of mental entities as well as identication of tangible entities in make-believe play give concrete shapes to shapeless thoughts and feelings. Such shaping is facilitated by the denial of seriousness. The above assertion, that make-believe play bypasses censorship, does not necessarily imply that what is realified in make-believe play is fully unconscious.

It has been argued that unconscious materials are coded in make-believe play as concrete symbols, which serve as a kind of disguise. It seems to me that a more accurate formulation would be based on the concept of an emotive's field of associations. What is realified are items belonging to this field. A suitable concrete entity can be identicated with such an item. The more peripheral the realified item, the less obvious is its association with the core of the emotive. This is an explication of the concept of symbol in this juncture. For example, the field of private associations surrounding the emotive of loneliness in the mind of a child can include ("symbolized as") being alone at home, a single camel in a desert and the moon in the dark sky. Each of these images can be realified in his play and represented with various objects identicated with it.

From Kindergarten age on, make-believe play becomes often less associative, more planned, organized and socialized and less influenced by the player's private images or by immediate environmental stimuli. The realified materials are more conventional, less private and idiosyncratic. For example, boys play at "battles between the good ones and the bad ones". Girls play at "Daddy, mommy and baby".

Fostering emotional wellness

Catharsis, abreaction

There are many non-play ways to release stress and tension and ease emotions such as sadness and anger – weeping, shouting, using violence on objects, people or animals, vigorous physical activities and more. Rough and tumble play, mock fighting, competitive sport games such as boxing matches that allow for legitimate, rule-governed uses of violence are also relatively harmless ways to release tensions and express emotions. Make-believe play facilitates ventilation of pent-up tensions and emotions in controlled, harmless manners, thanks to the denial of seriousness and the emotion-regulation techniques children use spontaneously in their play. For example, a boy can torture a doll representing a bully that has the habit of abusing him. One should not ignore the following considerations, however: (a) There are cases in which the expression of emotions such as anger and sadness in make-believe play does not have a cathartic, soothing effect but the opposite – increases and escalates the level of emotion arousal in an unstoppable feed-forward process. This happens when the emotions are particularly strong and when the player has not mastered the emotion-balancing techniques discussed in Chapter 11. (b) In some cases, despite the denial of seriousness, the player is frightened by the expression of his own emotions and falls into feelings of guilt, anxiety or shame. (c) In other cases, the players feign genuine cathartic expressions of emotions and tensions in their play without actually feeling them.

Positive emotions, counter-conditioning of fear, stress inoculation and stress management, resiliency

An assumption, almost taken for granted, is that play, being spontaneous, voluntary and free of constraints, is necessarily a fun-filled, joyful activity, incompatible with negative, stressful states of mind. Not necessarily so. Physical play and make-believe play can sometimes be effortful, competitive and frustrating. Often the affect accompanying play is not joy but curiosity, ambition to succeed and absorption in a specific, not necessarily cheerful or elated state of mind. Play can be calming and soothing with respect to past, present or anticipated stressful events, providing the players know how to activate its emotion-regulation functions. Otherwise the play can in some cases throw the player's emotions off-balance or even re-traumatize a traumatized player.

The emotion-regulation powers of make-believe play are derived from its above-mentioned therapeutic properties, namely owning and alienations, basic duality, arbitrariness of the signifier and possible worlds, as well as from the assortment of emotion-balancing techniques skilled children use in their play, as discussed in Chapter 11.

As often mentioned, one of the emotion-balancing properties of make-believe play is *miniaturing*. For example, a child who was abused by an adult can replay the abuse with small puppets she can manipulate. This makes the abusing figures less threatening. The victim can feel that she has some sense of mastery with respect to the memorized traumatic event.

The emotion-regulation powers of make-believe play facilitate the development of resiliency in the face of adverse, traumatic experiences.

Enhancing social relationships

Social competence, attachment and empathy

Make-believe play and other forms of play are not necessarily vehicles of interpersonal communication or catalysts of social competence. However, socially oriented and interpersonally skilled toddlers and children are naturally motivated to share their play with others. Play-sharing in turn is a major developer of social competence.

Simple playful interactions between toddler and caretaker, involving imitation, coordination of gestures and voice, enhance attachment.

Playful interactions with peers and notably sociodramatic play provide a platform for the development of a wide range of social skills, such as learning from others by modeling, turn-taking, conjoint planning of the play narrative and co-creating its means and contents.

In sociodramatic play, children learn to negotiate the rights of use of play objects and territories, techniques of joining play groups and gaining a social status, all while drawing on laws the children themselves have created. Sociodramatic play accelerates the development of empathy and pro-social attitude, because, during the conjoint creation of a narrative, each of the participants is supposed to understand and take into consideration the wishes, feelings and stories of the other participants and obey the children's own rules. However, as mentioned above, only children with basic social skills can profit from participating in this sophisticated form of play. Children who lack such skills need the mediation of a trained play therapist. (See Chapter 10.)

Increasing personal strength

Creative problem solving

Children who play skillfully attempt various solutions to technical difficulties they encounter in their attempts to create play means. They explore various verbal and non-verbal playful means to express themselves. They are adept at managing interpersonal conflicts by manipulating make-believe contents. Again, such skills are available to children who have mastered the art of play. (See Chapter 10.)

Moral development

The above-mentioned roles of play-sharing in developing social competence, attachment and empathy provide a platform for internalizing moral values and conduct rules in socially oriented, socially competent children. (See Chapter 10.)

Accelerated psychological development

This concept is too vague to allow a serious discussion. One can decide to interpret it as referring to the role of play in the development of ego, self and object. Presumably, one of the ways children internalize external human objects and make them an integral part their own selves is incorporating other people's behaviors in their own make-believe play. A child realifies behaviors of caretakers and other people and identicates his/her own behavior or the behavior of objects such as puppets with the realified materials, and in this way makes the realified behaviors his or her own. The play signifiers and signified contents represent various parts and features of one's self. (See Chapters 8–11.)

Self-regulation

Again, this concept can mean many things. Make-believe play can facilitate the regulation of emotions and behaviors in various ways. Therapeutic properties of play such as owning and alienation and possible worlds enable the players to transfer their out-of-control emotions and acting out to the realm of make-believe, while disowning them. (See Chapters 8–11.)

Self-control

Rough and tumble play, in humans and animals, requires inhibiting real aggressive impulses. The denial of seriousness property of make-believe play compels the player to suppress and inhibit really aggressive and impulsive drives and just pretend. The *enhancing social relationships* property discussed above requires the player to exercise an adequate level of self-control for the interpersonal play to succeed. (See Chapter 10.)

Self-esteem

All forms of play provide the players opportunities to try and rehearse various kinds of skills and competencies but can also be frustrating. The therapeutic properties of play (owning and alienation, basic duality, arbitrariness of the signifier and possible worlds) enable the player to realize strengths he/she has not materialized in real life, and, contrariwise, to show his/her weaknesses without compromising their self-esteem, because of the denial of seriousness.

Summary of chapter 12

One of the most important contributions to the development of play therapy as a profession has been the attempts to describe and explain the therapeutic powers of play. Schaefer and Drewes (2014) and their followers have been the first to integrate play theory and research with the applied art of play therapy. Their work is backed up by a huge amount of research evidence. In this chapter their work is re-examined with a view to make some suggestions at improvements. It is argued that in order to evaluate the validity of the hypotheses concerning the therapeutic powers of play, it is necessary to distinguish between play and non-play, between different kinds of play and between specific curative properties of each kind of play. Clear, rigorous, formal definitions and distinctions, which can be operationalized, are required. Such definitions and distinctions are proposed in Chapters 4–11. The types and subtypes of therapeutic powers of play proposed are listed and commented upon. Comments on the subtype *self-expression*, subsumed under the type *facilitating communication* allude to the linguistic peculiarities and the various expressive functions of make-believe play discussed in Chapters 4–11. The play bug-busters of basic duality, owning and alienation make it easier for the player to bypass censorship, to express forbidden or "crazy" thoughts and feelings that belong to the core or periphery of one's emotives. Comments on the subtype *access to the unconscious*, also subsumed under *facilitating communication* focus on the differences between free associations and dreams and make-believe play. It is suggested that instead of talking about access to the unconscious, it would be more accurate to say that make-believe play gives concrete shapes to shapeless thoughts and feelings. Symbolic coding in make-believe play is explicated as realifying a member of the field of associations surrounding an emotive.

The second type, *fostering emotional wellness* includes the subtypes of *catharsis* and *abreaction*. It is asserted that make-believe play facilitates ventilation of pent up tensions and emotions in controlled, harmless manners, thanks to the denial of seriousness and the play's emotion-regulation techniques. Cautioning notes refer to cases in which such ventilation does not have the cathartic effect but escalates the level of emotion arousal, to cases in which the denial of seriousness is weak and to cases in which emotions are not really felt by the player. Other subtypes are subsumed under *facilitating communication* are *positive emotions, counter-conditioning of fear, stress inoculation* and *stress management and resiliency*. It is argued that play is not always joyful. Play can be calming and soothing, providing the players know how to activate its emotion-regulation functions.

The third type is *enhancing social relationships*. It includes the subtypes *social competence, attachment* and *empathy*. It is stated that simple playful interactions between toddler and caretaker, involving imitation and coordination of gestures and voice, enhance attachment. Sociodramatic play provides a platform for the development of a wide range of social skills. However, only children with basic social skills can profit from participating in this sophisticated form of play.

The fourth type is *increasing personal strength*. A subtype is *creative problem solving*. It is asserted that this is manifested in players' attempts to solve technical difficulties, to experiment with various modes of communication and to manage interpersonal conflicts. Another subtype is *moral development*. It is asserted that the roles of play-sharing in developing social competence, attachment and empathy provide an arena for internalizing moral values. A third subtype is *accelerated psychological development*. This vague concept can be interpreted as referring to the role of play in the development of ego, self and object. One of the ways children internalize external human objects and make them an integral part their own selves is incorporating other people's behaviors in their own make-believe play. The play signifiers and signified contents represent various parts and features of one's self. A fourth subtype is *self-regulation*. It is stated that therapeutic properties of play, such as owning and alienation and possible worlds, enable the players to transfer their out-of-control emotions and acting-out to the realm of make-believe, while disowning them.

Self-control is the fifth subtype. Rough and tumble play, in humans and animals, requires inhibiting real aggressive impulses. The denial of seriousness property of make-believe play compels the player to suppress and inhibit really aggressive and impulsive drives and just pretend. The sixth and last subtype is *self-esteem*. All forms of play provide the players opportunities to try and rehearse various kinds of skills and competencies. The therapeutic properties of play enable the player to realize strengths that do not materialize in real life, and, contrariwise, to show their weaknesses without compromising their self-esteem, because of the denial of seriousness.

Assignments

Give your own examples of children's play that manifest the therapeutic powers of play listed in this chapter. Suggest play-therapeutic applications based on these examples. The examples can be found in your own observations or play and in your own play therapy practice. You may find such examples also in the various cases, examples and vignettes found in this book. Examples can also be found in documentations of children's play in the play research and play therapy literature. References are included in the following classified list of publications below.

A classified list of publications

The therapeutic powers of play

Ariel, S. (1992). *Strategic family play therapy*. Chichester, UK: Wiley.
Ariel, S. (2002). *Children's imaginative play: A visit to Wonderland*. Westport, CT: Praeger.
Klein, M. (1975). *The psycho-analysis of children*. (Original work published in 1932). New York, NY: Delacorte.
Schaefer, Ch.E and Drewes, A.A. (2013). *The therapeutic powers of play: 20 core agents of change*. Hoboken, NJ: Wiley.

Documentation of children's play

Axline, V.M. (2013). *Play therapy – The inner dynamics of childhood*. London, UK: Hesperides Press.
Cattanach, A. (1997). *Children's stories in play therapy*. London, UK: Jessica Kingsley.

Cattanach, A. (2002). *The story so far: The play therapy narratives*. London, UK: Jessica Kingsley.

Korngold, H. (2016). *Stories from child & adolescent psychotherapy: A curious space*. UK: Routledge.

Piaget, J. (1962). *Play, dreams and imitation in childhood*. Translated by C. Gattegno and F., Hodgston. London, UK: Routledge and Kegan Paul.

Part 4

Planning a multi-systemic play therapy

Chapter 13
Multi-systemic diagnostic evaluation

Interdisciplinary seminar

Shlomo: Therapy informed by the Diamond Model requires multi-systemic diagnostic evaluation. The case is viewed from both a synchronic and a diachronic perspective. Synchronically, we collect and analyze information that enables us to formulate semiotic, cybernetic information-processing programs that belong to all the internal and external subsystems that are relevant to the case. We identify and name bugs that invaded the programs, especially in times of drastic change or crisis, in which the programs' previous simplicity had been lost and bug-producing attempts to preserve partial simplicity are made. We identify emotive-related emotions that got out of balance and therefore energize the bugs. We sketch a multi-systemic developmental profile of each client, concentrating on lines and dimensions of development that are relevant to the case.

We have learned how to collect and analyze information of some of these types, obtained by observations of free make-believe play. Such observations are not the only sources of diagnostic information relevant to the case. Methods of getting and analyzing relevant information in other ways are presented in my other publications, e.g. Ariel (2002, 2018). I'll present a case treated by myself. Afterwards we'll try to construct together a multi-systemic diagnostic evaluation. I'm not going to share with you all the information I have about this case, but enough to illustrate the concepts and methods.

Case 13.1 Gad
Gad (8.3) was referred to therapy by his school. During the classes he was detached from the environment and was spending most of the time playing with toy trucks and cars that he brought from home. During breaks he would not go outside. He would continue to play with the toy vehicles. He was silent most of the time, was speaking very little. When the teacher addressed him, he would not respond. The children were afraid of him, because if someone had said something to him or about him, even with a good intention, he would respond by beating them up. He was large, strong, but overweight and clumsy.

My colleague Odeda, a developmental and rehabilitation psychologist, administered him a series of psychological and developmental tests. She also examined his medical history. She ruled out autism-spectrum disorder, including Asperger, intellectual disability or delayed language and speech development. She found metabolic dysfunction, under-developed gross motor skills, high sensory sensitivity and attention deficit disorder.

I had interviewed the parents before I met Gad. His mother, 38-year-old Esther, a large, vigorous woman, entered the room with energetic steps. Her husband, 40-year-old Benny, trailed after her, leaning on crutches. He sat down at some distance from her. During the case history interview she was the one who answered all the question, using a fluent, orderly, sometimes bookish style, showing off her knowledge of psychological terms and general education. When I addressed Benny, he sheepishly said, "Ask her." When I insisted to hear his own viewpoint, he would say in a faint voice, "She knows."

Here are some of the main things I heard from Esther:

"You might say I had no childhood. I was a parental child, had to take care of my two little brothers, do house chores. My father was primitive. There was no arguing with him. If you dared contradict him, two slaps and it was over. He tried to turn me into plasticine, succeeded to turn my mother into plasticine. She was a slave at home. I was a motherless child. She was so depressed and tired and helpless that she couldn't take care of the home and children and most of the burden fell on my own lean shoulders. If I had not taken those things upon myself, she would have paid a heavy price for neglecting the house and the children.

In elementary school I got low marks because I couldn't concentrate on my studies, but I liked to read books.

My so-called father didn't let me continue studying after elementary school. A girl shouldn't be too smart. If I had brought books from the library, he would return them and tell the librarian not let her lend me books.

Shlomo: I would have preferred not to use the word "primitive". I would use conservative, domineering.
Esther: If you say so. I didn't know it, but I was depressed. Clinical death. Until I was resurrected, around the age of fourteen. "If slavery is not wrong, nothing is wrong", Abe Lincoln. People throw books into the trash. Shame. I was picking them up and reading them in a public park. Old newspapers and magazines too. I read all the classics. Learned languages. English, French. I was spending most of the day out of home, alone in the park. I came back home when my father returned from work. He didn't know that I wasn't home. I stopped doing all the home chores and taking care of my brothers. And lo and behold! My mother turned out to be very capable of doing all these things!

At the age of 18 I completed my high school studies as an extern and started university. Education undergrad. I threw it in my father's face. I funded my studies on my own. A student during the day, a waitress at night. Belle de Nuit. I got out of touch with my parents almost completely. But then I stopped my studies. I met Benny and got married, not only but also to escape from the prison called "home". I was 21 then. Benny worked as a truck driver. He had a job. Could bring bread home, Just bread. We bought an apartment with blood, sweat and tears. I didn't fall in love, but what is love? "Love is as smoke", *Romeo and Juliet*.

(She continued, failing to notice the sad, agonized look on Benny's face.)

I didn't want to be a slave at home like my mother. I was rational. He's a good man. Calm. Pure soul. I couldn't fall in love anyway. An extinct volcano. I would have to shed dozens of shells from myself to reach the fire and lava core. I couldn't do it then. Maybe in the future. I stopped my formal studies, also because I wanted to be a perfect, full-time mother. I continue reading and learning at home, an autodidact. My mother offered to help. I didn't want her help and I didn't let the man who had inseminated my mother approach my boy.

I sent Gad to kindergarten only at the age of five. I flooded him with toys and books. I compensated him for what I had missed in childhood. It's difficult for me to accept that Gad is only interested in cars and trucks. I made a law that he had to read a book for 15 minutes every evening before bedtime. But I know my boy. Deep inside he is very intelligent and intellectually curious. He is post-traumatic, because of the accident. Closed up. At the end of the summer vacation, just before Gad entered second grade, we travelled in the mountains, in my husband's van. He ran into a traffic barrier. The car overturned. Miraculously, we stayed alive, but my husband hit a rock and broke the pelvic bones. Since then he has been 70 percent disability. We live on National Insurance and from odd jobs I do, baby-sitting, cleaning apartments and stuff. I have no choice, I must let my mother take care of Gad when I'm not at home. My father sometimes stays with her in my home and plays with Gad. I don't like it. When I'm not at work I tell him to go home.

Shlomo: I asked Esther, "What about the recommendations Odeda wrote in the diagnostic reports?"

Esther: I haven't done anything with it yet. I can't find the time.

Observation 13.1 A family free play session

Esther is sitting at one corner of the room and Benny at another corner. Gad, without saying a word and without looking at his father, at his mother or at me, takes a large selection of toy cars from a drawer and throws them on the carpet in the middle of the room. He builds a high wall of play blocks around one of the cars, a black one. The rest of the cars he piles about two meters from the wall, some turned upside down.

Esther and Benny were instructed before the meeting to try to join Gad's play as play partners.

Esther takes an old woman's doll, sits down on the carpet near Gad and says, as if from the mouth of the doll, "I'm your driving instructor, may I come in? The driving lesson is about to begin."

Gad ignores her. He takes more play blocks and begins building a second layer of wall around the wall he had built.

Benny looks at a loss. He asks Esther, "What should I do?" Then he turns his gaze to me. Esther tells him to "play with cars". He gets up with difficulty, leaning on his crutches, hobbling to a toy truck at the end of the room. He sits down and starts moving the truck forward and backward with one of his crutches.

Gad makes an opening in the double wall of blocks, on the side of the wall that doesn't face Esther. He takes the black car out through the opening and starts driving it toward the room's wall, away from Esther and Benny.

Esther says, "Oh, I see you're ready for the driving lesson!" He ignores her. He accelerates the car's speed, moving it round and round in circles.

Esther says, "You are so advanced in your driving skills that now you are driving a racing car. I'm driving a racing car, too. Let's see who wins." She moves her car in circles parallel to Gad's car. He pulls his car away from her and moves it toward the wall. He makes the car climb the wall with lightning speed, moving it in circles on the wall. Esther says, "Be careful, this mountain road is very steep! I don't want you to fall!"

Gad moves the car down to the carpet, heading toward his father. Benny bends down and drives the truck toward Gad's car, causing a head-on collision. Gad takes Benny's truck, walks toward the pile of cars and throws the truck on the pile, upside down. He enters his black car to the enclosed space surrounded by blocks and closes the opening with two blocks.

Shlomo: OK, let's try to construct a multi-systemic diagnostic evaluation on the basis of the admittedly limited information that we have.

Let's begin with a diachronic analysis. It will necessarily be based on Esther's answers in the case history interview, yes, subjective, but be that as it may. First, we'll try to identify the relevant internal and external programs at every stage in the history of the case.

Anna: Of each of the people involved?
Shlomo: Yes, and also their inter-relationships programs.
Ethan: Relevant to what?
Shlomo: Relevant to the current situation, synchronically.
Daniel: If I understand what you mean by stages, then I would divide the history of the case into the following stages: Stage 1 – Esther's childhood until she was 14; Stage 2 – her teenage years, until she was 18, when she began rebelling against her father's control, but without confronting him directly; Stage 3 – 18 to 21, her unfinished university years, in which she rebelled against her father openly; Stage 4 – her marriage and Gad's birth, until the accident, when Gad was six, just before he entered second grade; Stage 5 – the period

of the family's coping with the aftermath of the accident, until the beginning of therapy, when Gad was in second grade.

Shlomo: I don't think I would have divided this history into periods in a different way. Let us now look at the main external and internal programs we can identify in each period, including the relevant characteristics of the developmental profile of each of the actors in this drama, to the extent that we have data that allow us to obtain such a picture. We should also try to identify bugs in the various programs in each stage. More specifically, let's look at losses of previous simplicity in each stage and bug-producing, deviation-amplifying attempts to restore partial simplicity at the times of transition between the stages.

Lailah: And if we don't have such data?

Shlomo: Then and in any other cases the results of our analyses will be hypotheses, to be confirmed or refuted when we have more data.

Let's recall. The internal subsystems (within the individual) are: The body (the brain and the nervous system, the genetic, anatomic and physiological subsystems); the cognitive and psychomotor subsystems; conscious or unconscious emotional concerns, emotional conflicts and emotional defenses; the individual and social personality (self and body images and concepts, object relations, self and body boundaries, attachment, egocentricity and narcissism vs. empathy and prosocial attitude, reality testing, self-control, psychosexual development, moral development; the internalized culture, etc.). The external subsystems are: Significant life events; the family and other social systems; the ecosystems (the human and nonhuman environment at large) and the culture.

The developmental parameters are: Growth; internalization; complexity; coordination and integration; differentiation; depth of processing; concreteness vs. abstraction; constancy and stability; flexibility; objectivity; monitoring and control; socialization.

Lailah: I believe that analyzing the internal programs of Esther's father and mother would not be relevant to understanding and dealing with the current situation. What is important is Esther's family relationships, which had shaped those parts of her personality that were reflected in the current situation. Based on the partial and subjective information at our disposal concerning the first stage of the case history, I can say that I don't see in Esther's father any proximity goals with respect to his wife and daughter, only control goals, which were motivated by his cultural norms and personality. Esther's control goal with respect to her father was to obey him and let him control her. Her plan included not provoking him in any manner, not showing her strengths, emotions, wishes and needs. Her control goal with respect to her mother was to protect her from her father. Her plan included interpreting her mother's input as proof that she could not meet her husband's demands and taking upon herself to fulfill these demands.

Ethan: I think her control programs were infected with the bug horse blinders, because she withheld from her parents (and from the school too) information about her real strengths, about who she really was. Do the term horse blinders apply to the output of one's programs?

Shlomo: Yes, to every stage of the processing.

Ethan: Her main emotive was fear of her father's threatening, punitive personality and physical violence. Her horse blinders were a defense against this emotive.

Anna: In terms of cognitive development, she was at least within the limits of her age norms, despite her low achievements in school, because she was not emotionally available to study. I don't think we have enough information to obtain a more complete and accurate profile of her cognitive development or to analyze her profile according to the developmental parameters in the list. Maybe it would be correct to say that her self-concept, in so far as her cognitive abilities are concerned, was infected with horse blinders.

Shlomo: The very fact that you can put your finger on the kinds of information we lack and to formulate the information in the terminology you have learned is important for our purposes.

Daniel: OK. Considering the fact that we lack a lot of information, we can speculate that her bugged control programs and her emotive compelled her to develop a high level of self-control (the monitor and control parameter). She also had to relinquish the egocentricity and narcissism appropriate for her age and develop empathy toward her mother and, at least on the surface, a pro-social attitude, beyond what is expected of a girl her age. In terms of the developmental parameters I think I would refer to growth, differentiation, monitoring and control and socialization.

Lailah: To continue speculating, I am asking myself what can be said about her internalized objects and about her self-concept. It seems that at that stage she internalized the person of her mother as she conceived it. I recall her extremely powerful expressions, "I was depressed, clinical death."

Anna: These expressions struck me like lightning.

Lailah: And she internalized the image of a domineering man, who does not see women as human beings with needs, wishes and rights. In terms of the developmental parameters, I would refer to a low level of complexity. She had a simplistic image of her parents (due to the horse blinders bug, she based her judgement on limited information). Therefore, her level of internalization was also low. I would say also, a low level of differentiation. It has to do with self and body boundaries. Also, she wanted to protect her mother. She could not fully differentiate herself from her mother, as she conceived her. A low level of objectivity in this respect.

Shlomo: An interesting analysis.

Anna: What about attachment? She could not get attached to her father.

Ethan: Maybe at that state she internalized some aspects of his culture concerning the roles of women.

Anna: She was attached to her mother, but on a low level of differentiation.

Shlomo: OK, let's go to the second stage, Esther's teenage years.

Daniel: The simplicity of Stage 1 was lost. Her proximity goal was now to keep distance from both her parents. Her plan was simply spending as little time at home as she could. Her control goal with respect to her father was not to let him control her. Her plan was to do what she wanted, mainly reading, away from his intrusive and supervising eyes, but not to confront him directly. Her control goal with respect to her mother was simply not being available to fulfil any duties imposed on her. Her mother co-operated.

Ethan: In terms of loss of simplicity, in Esther's proximity and control plans, as well as in her mother's proximity and control plans, I see mainly a loss of comprehensiveness and loss of consistency. Her having stayed out of home all day and reading books were data that didn't exist before. All day she stayed out of home, and when her father was home, she behaved as if nothing changed. This is inconsistent. The way I see it, she preferred plausibility at the cost of comprehensiveness and consistency. She interpreted the input from her father and mother more correctly than before and could make more plausible predictions. She understood that her father cannot have full control over her and that her mother is not so helpless. She was less afraid and angrier. She developed a new emotive – anger at her own and her mother's weakness and at her father's aggression.

Anna: Do you mean to say that at this stage she had the bugs horse blinders and flip-flop?

Ethan: Yes.

Anna: What kinds of information did she miss?

Ethan: For instance, that she could confront her father directly. She realized that only when she reached Stage 3. She also missed the possibility of getting close to her mother.

Shlomo: Good thinking. Her bugs kept her farther away from her mother and prevented her from getting from her mother corrective feedback that would let them create a new positive mother-daughter relationship. Feed-forward, amplified deviation from hemostasis.

Lailah: If we look at Esther's cognitive and self-concept programs, at this stage her general knowledge and cognitive skills grew considerably. She began to internalize a self-concept of a knowledgeable, intelligent person with an insatiable thirst for knowledge. She got rid of her previous horse blinders bug concerning her cognitive abilities.

Anna: This was also a defensive reaction against her father having prohibited her to learn and develop, and a rebellion against his cultural norms.

Daniel: It appears that at this stage Esther further developed her self-boundary on the differentiation parameter, but regressed in empathy, pro-social attitude and attachment. She didn't let herself internalize her mother as an attachment figure.

Shlomo: OK, third stage.

Lailah: Proximity goal with respect to her father and mother – to increase the distance between them and herself, almost totally cutting off their relationships. Plan – not being available, too busy.

Control goal with respect to her father – full release from his control. Plan – to act openly, without fear, against his will and cultural norms, to be independent financially.

Ethan: Loss of simplicity? Loss of comprehensiveness. In her previous plans, the input from her father and his responses were something to be considered and beware of. No more. Her goals and plans with respect to her parents at this stage were motivated by despair of the possibility of having their understanding and support. That was her main emotive then.

Daniel: To restore simplicity partially, she preferred consistency (consistent independence and lack of contact with parents) at the cost of comprehensiveness (not considering the possibility of building a new type of relationship with her parents, appropriate to her not being a minor anymore) and parsimony (ignoring the possibility that the past relationships were no longer relevant to the present) – horse blinders and fifth wheel.

Lailah: One can say that the effects on the development of her personality were like in the previous phase, only strengthened and stabilized.

Shlomo: Next stage. Esther's marriage and Gad's birth.

Ethan: It seems to me that at that stage the rebellion against her parents had been completed. Because of the alienation from them, living with them as strangers under the same roof, all devoted just to her studies, she began to feel loneliness and emptiness. This was her new emotive. Her need to find a partner, to leave her parents' home and to raise her own family was stronger than her will to complete her university studies. In terms of loss of simplicity, her previous stage programs lost their relevance. They also lost their comprehensiveness, because they didn't cover her new needs. She preferred parsimony (developing new programs that are more relevant to her present life stage) and consistency (developing interpersonal programs that do not include a conflict between her allegiance to her family of origin and devotion to a new partner and family) at the expense of comprehensiveness (finding a way to reconcile a different and renewed relationship with her family of origin with a new relationship with a partner). Horse blinders.

Anna: In terms of the developmental parameters, I see a resumed growth of attachment needs, but not attachment to her parents.

Lailah: I'm not sure I agree with you, Ethan and Anna. Esther didn't look for someone to love. She declared that she didn't marry Benny out of love and that she wasn't capable of loving. I would say that her attachment ability was impaired. In terms of depth of processing, her feelings for other people and having empathy were shallow. We saw this in the interview and in the family play. She didn't notice Benny's sad facial expression when she said she didn't fall in love with him. In the play session she didn't sit close to Benny and didn't try to involve him in the play. The roles she played were "a driving teacher" and "a racing cars competitor". She forced Gad to read books and had difficulty accepting his choice to play with cars.

I think her main motivation to marry and raise a child was to compensate herself not for the lack of love but for her childhood, in which she was controlled by her father, served as a parental child and was invisible as a person.

Daniel: Let us consider the reasons for her choice of Benny – a way to leave the parents' home, in which she felt imprisoned; finding a breadwinner that will allow her to devote herself to raising the child and reading books. In a way, she wanted to return to her childhood role in her parents' home, to take care of the home and the child, but by choice, not by coercion. She preferred a person who is less educated than her, less verbal, weaker, not dominant, whom she could control.

With respect to Benny she had a control goal. I didn't see a proximity goal. Her plan was to impose on him the burden of earning a living, without being interested in him personally. Her plan was infected with horse blinders and non-sense. She was unaware of his emotional needs, of his difficulty in accepting her lack of emotional attachment to him. She also interpreted his silence as an expression of absence of such emotional needs.

Shlomo: And what about Benny's goals and plans with respect to Esther?

Daniel: On the face of it, it looks as if he had only a control goal, wanting her to control him, but I believe he had mainly a proximity goal with respect to her. He wanted her to love him and accept him. Letting her control him seems to be a part of his plan to achieve his proximity goal, not an end in itself. His plan was not to provoke her in any way, not to show her who he really is, not to have an impact, lest she put him down and reject him.

Anna: My question is, was his difficulty in expressing himself verbally indicative of a low level of cognitive and linguistic development, on the parameters of complexity and concreteness vs. abstraction? Or was it a product of a low self-esteem, which in the relationship with Esther had only been exacerbated? Daniel, you said, "not to show her who he really was." But who was he, really? Did he wear horse blinders that prevented him from seeing and showing his real self or was what he showed his real self?

Shlomo: An important question in terms of the therapeutic approach. We have to consider the limit of our expectations of him.

Lailah: Daniel, I found what you said about Esther's urge to return to her role in the parents' home in childhood interesting. Indeed, she devoted the first five years of Gad's life totally to raising him and do house chores. Where had her desire to be free gone?

Ethan: In a way, this looks like repetition compulsion. She internalized a certain role and couldn't really get rid of it, had to regress there.

Daniel: I think she had a proximity goal with respect to Gad, but not proximity in the sense of attachment and pure love. She herself said that she compensated him for what she had missed in her own child. Mainly flooded him with books and toys. She projected on him her own narcissistic needs. Her plan to achieve this proximity goal was to keep him close to herself for five years, and also to have him exclusively to herself, not letting anybody else get really close to him, nursery schools, baby sitters, her parents, his father, professional helpers, educators.

Ethan: That was also a control goal. She wanted to shape him to become a duplicate of her own ideal self and didn't trust anybody else to interfere. She also wanted to protect him against her own father. I think both her proximity and control plans with respect to him were infected with horse blinders, non-sense and fifth wheel. Her own childhood experiences were irrelevant to his developmental needs. Her parents were not necessarily the same as when they had raised her, and she did not take into account the fact that Gad needed more people besides her, including grandparents. She said that deep inside he was very intelligent and intellectually curious. This was a projective identification, projecting on him her own self as a child that did not show her intellectual assets. She didn't acknowledge his real limitations and shortcomings.

Lailah: Gad instinctively felt the bugs in her plans for proximity and control with respect to himself. His proximity and control goals were to protect himself against her intrusiveness and her attempts to dominate him. We saw this clearly in the family play – surrounding his toy car, which apparently signified himself, by an impenetrable wall, a double wall; ignoring her attempts to join his play; and moving his car away from her.

Ethan: We lack data on the relationship between Gad and his father. The only evidence of the connection between them was when Gad moved his car in the direction of his father, and Benny caused a collision between his truck and Gad's car. It's a kind of contact. As we saw, Gad avoided any connection between his car and his mother's, and here he initiated a contact with his father.

Anna: Benny was a truck driver before the accident. Gad's obsessive play with toy trucks and cars was perhaps his way of identifying with his father.

Daniel: Then Gad took the toy truck, walked toward the pile of cars he had created and threw the truck on the pile upside down. I think the collision was a symbolic representation of the accident. The pile represented a junkyard for wrecked vehicles. It seems to me that throwing Benny's truck on the pile stood for referring to his disabled father as a damaged, useless good.

Anna: Not just because of his handicap, also because of his passivity. Gad was ambivalent with respect to his father. He wanted to get close to him, but realized that his proximity goal couldn't be reached. There was tremendous anger in this act of throwing the truck over the pile.

Lailah: Maybe Gad's proximity plan with respect to Benny was infected with horse blinders and non-sense. Maybe he didn't realize that Benny was not as damaged or useless as he believed.

Shlomo: We'll return to this question later, when we discuss the last stage, after the accident. OK, Stage 5, Gad's school years and the accident.

Lailah: I think the main development at this stage was Esther's being compelled to face Gad's academic, social and behavioral difficulties in the kindergarten and in the first two years of school. Ethan said (I wrote down everything) that Esther wanted to shape Gad to become a duplicate of her own ideal self. He also said that her claim that deep inside Gad was very intelligent and intellectually curious was a projective identification, projecting on him her own self as a child who didn't show her intellectual assets. Ethan said that she didn't acknowledge Gad's real limitations and shortcomings. But in school these limitations and shortcomings were floating to the surface.

Daniel: Nor did she understand that her having kept him alone with her at home couldn't but adversely affect his social development.

Ethan: We can relate to this stage as a phase of loss of simplicity. The input from his school performance was new information, previously unavailable to her former internalized image of Gad. A loss of comprehensiveness.

Shlomo: We can reformulate what you said in information-processing terms but let's not do it now.

Daniel: Based on our data, Esther did not completely ignore the difficulties, but attributed them to the lack of externalization of Gad's inner personality, just as she had not externalized her own inner personality as a child.

Lailah: This disappointment was unbearable. Bugs are energized by unbalanced emotions. She chose to forgo parsimony (sticking to her previous image of Gad, which was no longer valid), comprehensiveness (refusing to see the whole picture of Gad's functioning) and plausibility (misinterpreting his behavior) to preserve consistency (a consistent image of Gad as having an inner personality like her own). Fifth wheel, non-sense and horse blinders.

Anna: We decided that Gad was defective, but the diagnosis found no intellectual disability or delayed language and speech development. So maybe she was not so wrong?

Shlomo: You are right. All our hypotheses should be considered tentative, until we have further confirming or disconfirming evidence.

Anna: Maybe his lack of talk was elective mutism? Maybe he identified with his father's preference not to talk?

Shlomo: Maybe. Odeda's diagnosis ruled out autism spectrum disorder, including Asperger. She found metabolic dysfunction, under-developed gross motor skills, over-sensitivity and attention deficit disorder.

Anna: He inherited from his mother her large, strong body.

Lailah: The metabolic dysfunction was responsible for his being overweight. The under-developed gross motor skills made him clumsy. Because of the over-sensitivity, he shut himself off from powerful stimuli. The ADD caused him distractions. He found it hard to listen and participate in class activities. To overcome this, he occupied himself obsessively with his favorite play.

Daniel: All these limitations prevented him from participating in sports activities and rough and tumble games. All these, together with the lack of social skills because of the forced separation from company in his early years, caused him to shut himself within himself, avoid the other children and fail to function as a pupil.

Anna: In his play we saw both this seclusion (encircling his truck in the walls) and make-believe compensation for his limitations – a truck that's running fast like a racing car and climbs walls that seem to signify steep mountains.

Ethan: His proximity goal was to avoid proximity. His plan was not to communicate verbally, not to participate in any activity, concentrating on his play with cars, staying inside the class during breaks, etc. This plan was infected with horse blinders, because he filtered out any information that would have allowed him to get feedback from the environment and had not considered any other possibility to deal with his difficulties.

Lailah: His sensitivity to the children's behavior toward him indicates narcissism, but because of the low level of social skills, the seclusion and lack of use of the verbal medium, he responded with physical aggression. One can say that this was his plan to serve his control goal of not being controlled by his peers, but the plan was infected with non-sense and horse blinders. He responded with physical violence even when children tried to relate to him positively and did not take into account his own contribution to the negative attitude towards him.

Shlomo: OK. The accident and what followed.

Daniel: That was a crisis that led to the loss of simplicity of previous programs. Before that, it was clear that Benny was the one who worked and provided for the family and Esther stayed at home. After the accident Benny was the one who stayed at home and Esther was the one who had to provide for the family. She had to do simple jobs that didn't fit her self-image as an intelligent and talented woman. Before the accident Benny had been healthy. After the accident he was crippled. These are facts that had not been in the family's proximity and control programs before the accident. Loss of comprehensiveness. Also, loss of parsimony, because some of the previous facts were no longer relevant to the new situation.

Ethan: This could have been an opportunity for Benny to get closer to Gad and to be more dominant in relation to him (proximity/control goals) but Benny did not take advantage of this opportunity and put himself in an even more marginal place. Horse blinders, because it didn't occur to him that he could form a new kind of relationship with his son.

Anna: His low self-image became even lower. Gad, who in the past had not internalized him as a significant masculine parental role model, began to see him as a worthless object, total loss, as expressed in his play, throwing the truck on the pile of scrap vehicles. Gad's plan was also infected with horse blinders and non-sense, because Benny wasn't really insignificant and could develop his parental skills despite his disability. He could go through a process of rehabilitation, personally and professionally. Gad should not reject him. Because Esther wasn't home all the time, Gad was free of her pressure.

Ethan: Naturally, the accident had a traumatic effect on the entire family. Esther seemed to be trying to maintain a partial simplicity. She gave up comprehensiveness, failed to take into account all the new data. She also gave up parsimony, recognition that the past was no longer fully relevant to the new situation, but attempted to consistently keep the past frozen. She kept Benny in his marginal position, preferred not to acknowledge Gad's difficulties, including the impact of the accident on him, and even ignored the impact of the accident on herself, on her self-image and on the entire family. Horse blinders and fifth wheel.

Shlomo: Let's try to do a componential analysis (CDCA) of Gad's play in the observation (Table 13.1), without going to all the steps of the analysis, just use your logic, intuition and creativity to draw the final chart.

(Anna, Lailah, Daniel and Ethan start working).

Lailah: OK, this is the result we have reached. Main emotive: Fear of being weak and vulnerable.

Shlomo: Excellent. We can see the emotion-balancing dynamics of his play. He started by feeling weak, vulnerable, penetrable, and protected himself by a wall. When his mother tried to invade his personal space, he fortified the wall with another wall. Then when he felt safe, he went out and started moving, faster and faster, alone, feeling powerful and impenetrable. Then he felt safe enough to approach his father, but when the latter caused his truck to crash into his son's truck, Gad felt insecure again. He recalled the accident and his father's disability. He threw his father's truck on the pile, far away from his own truck, and entered again into the space surrounded by walls.

In play-therapeutic work with Gad, we can activate these emotion-balancing mechanisms together.

Anna: I feel overwhelmed, so much information!

Shlomo: Let's collect our findings and list them: Emotives, developmental profiles, proximity-controls goals and plans and bugs in the various programs. We'll describe them from a synchronic perspective. This list will serve as a basis for building an initial, tentative therapeutic strategy.

Anna: But we said that many of our findings were speculative, based on a very limited range of data.

Shlomo: Most enterprises start with strategies or plans that are based on limited and often speculative data, e.g. business enterprises, military operations,

Table 13.1 Semantic CDCA of Observation 13.1 (Gad)

The intensity of fear	High	Medium	Low
Subdimensions			
Inside vs. a protected space	inside, surrounded by impenetrable wall;	opening the wall; Starts going out; pile of scrap vehicles;	out in the open air;
Speed of movement	no movement;	slow movement;	fast movement;
Movement direction	horizontal;		vertical;
Closeness to vehicles	close;	not so close;	far, unreachable;
Condition of Vehicle	total loss, on pile;		good condition;

football games, etc. The initial strategy keeps changing according to the terrain condition and the new data that stream in.

(The participants start preparing the list.)

Daniel: OK, here is the list. We added a few things that we haven't discussed so far.

Shlomo: Excellent!

Daniel: Emotives and emotional conflicts, and developmental profiles:

Benny – shame and feelings of inferiority; feeling weak, unintelligent, insecure, useless. Guilt for having caused the accident; mourning for the loss of his good physical condition and work ability; shame for not being able to provide for his family.

As for his developmental profile, we asked ourselves whether his difficulty in expressing himself verbally was indicative of a low level of cognitive and linguistic development or a product of low self-esteem. We didn't have a conclusive answer. If the latter, then programs related to his self are infected with horse blinders.

Esther – fear of not being appreciated, of not being visible, of being controlled and effaced as a person; anger at her parents, mourning her lost childhood; frustration that she is forced to work in jobs that do not reflect her potential; sadness at the loss of her husband as provider; frustration that she had to accept her mother as a caretaker for Gad and her father's presence in his life.

With respect to her developmental profile, we hypothesized that since her adolescence she developed her self-boundaries and regressed in empathy and pro-social attitude. She didn't let herself internalize her mother as an attachment figure. Her attachment ability was impaired.

Gad – shame and feelings of inferiority because of his physical limitations; fear of being exposed to derision and mockery; fear and anger at attempts to force him to be and act against his will and preferences and beyond his abilities.

In terms of the developmental parameters, Odeda found no intellectual disability or delayed language and speech development. We asked ourselves whether he had a mild form of elective mutism or rather identified with his father's preference not to talk. But he had metabolic dysfunction and under-developed motor skills, over-sensitivity and ADD. All these impaired his development in the academic, physical and social spheres. He also had not internalized his father as a role model.

Shlomo: As I said, bugs are energized by emotive-related unbalanced emotions. So, removing or weakening the bugs requires finding ways of restoring the emotional balance. This can be done by play therapy, as we learned in our previous sessions. Both emotives and bugs are related also to the developmental profiles of the clients. Let's embed the emotives and developmental profiles in the right places in the proximity-control goals and plans, and in the bugs in the plans. We will also identify bugs in programs that are not interpersonal.

Ethan:

Esther with respect to Gad:

Control goals:
>To mold him in the shape of her own ideal self. To protect him from external influences.

Plan:
>If she has no choice but to involve others in his upbringing, minimize such involvement.
>
>If he does not behave according to her goal, interpret it as just a superficial external expression and try to force him to co-operate partially, like reading every day.

Bugs:

Fifth wheel: Her own ideal self and past experiences are irrelevant to his personality and current life.
>Developmentally, she differentiated herself from her parents, but could not differentiate herself from Gad. Fifth wheel.
>
>The emotive that energized this bug was mourning for her lost childhood.

Horse blinders: She didn't take into account that minimizing the involvement of others in his upbringing was contrary to her goal, because it prevents him from acquiring the knowledge and skills that could bring him closer to her ideal self.
>This bug is energized by her fear of being controlled and effaced as a person and by her frustration that she had to accept her mother as a caretaker for Gad and her father's presence in his life.
>
>Developmentally, this has to do with her egocentricity and regressed pro-social attitude.

Non-sense: Failing to realize that what she sees is perhaps what she gets, that Gad's behavior reflects his real preferences and limitations and there is no depth underneath them.
>This bug is energized by projecting on Gad her fear of not being appreciated, of being effaced as a person. This bug is also energized by mourning her lost childhood. She couldn't accept that Gad was effaced as a person too, and that she was to be blamed.

Horse blinders: Ignoring the fact that the pressure she was exerting on Gad only made him resist. This bug is also energized by the same emotives.

Proximity goal:
>Keep Gad close to herself in her own terms.

Plan:
>Getting close to him physically and trying to engage him in verbal and non-verbal communication, without warmth or real intimacy.
>
>If he moves away from her and does not respond, she continues to try.

Bugs:
Horse blinders: She didn't realize that what he really needed was warmth and intimacy. She didn't consider other kinds of relationship with Gad.

Developmentally, this bug was influenced also by her impaired attachment ability.

She didn't take into account that the attempts to approach him in her own way only kept him away from her.

Anna:
Gad with respect to Esther:
Proximity and control Goals:
Not letting Esther control him and not letting her get close to him.
Plan:
If Esther is trying to get close to me and instruct me, I do not respond. If she insists I either create a physical barrier between me and her or increase the distance between us.

Bugs:
Horse blinders: He didn't realize that avoiding her increased her anxiety and frustration and caused her to try harder. He didn't consider other ways to express his resistance, that would perhaps help her and him develop a new kind of relationship.

This bug was energized by the emotive fear and anger at attempts to force him to be and act against his will and preferences, and beyond his abilities.

Developmentally these goals and plan had to do with his over-sensitivity and other limitations.

Lailah:
Benny with respect to Gad:
Proximity and control goals:
Not to get close to Gad and neither control him nor being controlled by him.
Plan:
Not to initiate physical or verbal contact with Gad, unless told to, or unless Gad would initiate the contact.

Bugs:
Horse blinders: Benny was unaware of the fact that Gad would have wanted for the two of them to be closer to each other, providing Benny had shown a wish to have such closer relationships and to be more present and more dominant.

This bug was energized by the emotives of shame and feeling inferior and useless; guilt for the accident, thinking he was not entitled to be a parent.

Gad with respect to Benny:
Proximity and control goals:
Neither to control Benny, nor to be controlled by him. To explore the possibility of creating a certain degree of closeness between them.
Plan:
Get close to Benny and test his response. Challenge him to be more dominant and more present, by showing him that he is not.

Bug:
Horse blinders: He did not see that this challenge, like showing Benny that he was handicapped, could only discourages Benny.
Emotives: Ashamed of his father, anger at his weakness.
Developmentally: Lack of internalization of a male identification figure.
Daniel:
Esther with respect to Benny:
Control goal:
> To control him.

Plan:
> Not trying to urge him to be more present, more dominant and more active as a partner and as a parent.

Bugs:
Horse blinders: She didn't consider the possibility that if she gave him more presence and a more central place, she and Gad would also benefit from it.
Emotives: Fear of being controlled; sadness at his loss as provider.
Developmentally: Impaired attachment and empathy ability.
Proximity goal:
> To be present but not too close.

Plan:
> To have him around but not initiate any kind of intimacy.

Bugs:
> Horse blinders and non-sense.
> She misinterpreted his passivity as indicating no need for intimacy and warmth.
> Maybe she felt anger at his disability, without blaming him consciously.

Developmentally: Impaired attachment ability and empathy.
Benny with respect to Esther:
Proximity and control goals:
> To be controlled by her and preserve some degree of proximity.

Plan:
> Avoid expressing his wishes, needs and opinions. Letting her talk about and for him too, instead of talking about and for himself.

Bug:
Horse blinders: He predicted that if he would be more dominant, she would put him down and not want him.
Emotive: Feeling useless. His only worth was as a provider, otherwise he believed he was not entitled to have a position of a husband and father.
Lailah:
Esther with respect to her mother (related to Gad):
Control goal:
> Minimizing her mother's involvement as a caretaker, to prevent her mother from influencing Gad with her weakness, passivity and lack of intellect.

Proximity goal:
> Minimizing contact, admitting her mother just as a babysitter.

Emotives: Frustration that she had to accept her mother as a caretaker for Gad. Frustration that she had to work in idiot jobs; anger at her parents and at her lost childhood.
Bugs:
Fifth wheel: Her childhood experience with her mother wasn't relevant to her functioning as a grandmother.
Horse blinders: Being blind to the benefits for Gad of his grandmother participating in his upbringing.
Developmental: Differentiation from parents endangered.
Esther with respect to her father (related to Gad):
Control goal:
    Not to let him control Gad.
Proximity goal:
    Minimizing contact.
Bug: Fifth wheel, his having controlled her in the past was irrelevant to his present relationship with Gad.
Shlomo: Anna, I hope you are less overwhelmed. It is true that even when we concentrated the data, we still have a large quantity of difficult materials. But in the multi-systemic approach we learn, it is impossible to simplify the picture further. What we have gathered here will serve as a basis for us to build an initial strategy.

Summary of chapter 13

Therapy informed by the Diamond Model requires multi-systemic diagnostic evaluation. The case is viewed from both a synchronic and a diachronic perspective. The diagnostic evaluation includes formulations of semiotic, cybernetic information-processing programs belonging to all those internal and external subsystems that are relevant to the case. Bugs in these programs are identified and named. The same applies to emotive-related emotions that got out of balance and therefore energized the bugs. A multi-systemic developmental profile of each client is sketched, concentrating on lines and dimensions of development that are relevant to the case. It is advisable to organize all of this information in short lists or in a tabular form, in order to make it easier to refer to these data when we plan therapeutic strategies.

Assignments

Write a multi-systemic diagnostic evaluation of the following case:

Case 13.2 Bassel
Eight-year-old Bassel was rejected by his school peers. He used to bully his classmates, threaten the teachers and from time to time run away

from school. At home, he suffered from fears. He would demand his stepmother Yasmina to stay with him in the bathroom. He refused to sleep in his own bed and was sneaking into his father and Yasmina's bed. Along with that, however, he would not let Yasmina get close to him emotionally, touch or hug him. He would call her names and insult her.

From birth Bassel had suffered from metabolic imbalance. He was overweight, low on gross motor skills, slow, breathing heavily, getting tired easily and having difficulties running and climbing. However, he was big and strong. Because of his emotional and social difficulties, he could not realize his full potential as a pupil.

Bassel was the only child of 40-year-old Zacharia, a Muslim Arab, who was usually unemployed, but had occasional odd jobs in the street market or in construction. Bassel's biological mother, Rodica, was a foreign worker from Romania. She committed suicide due to postpartum depression when Bassel was six-months-old. Half a year after Rodica's death, Zacharia married Yasmina, a Muslim Arab. At the onset of therapy Yasmina was pregnant.

The family lived in a small town, inhabited by Muslim Arabs and Jews, near Tel Aviv, in a low socioeconomic area.

Bassel was referred to the community mental health outpatient clinic by the local authority's social service. Lamar, a clinical social worker, oversaw the case. I served as her supervisor.

Lamar interviewed Zacharia and Yasmina and got the following sketchy history of the case:

Zacharia, Bassel's father, grew up in a traditional Muslim family of a lower-middle socioeconomic status. As a child, Zacharia didn't like studying and was associating with children who tended toward delinquency. His father used to beat him up to discipline him. His mother was submissive and did not protect him, but she loved him.

Zacharia's father had a successful garage that got into financial difficulty when Zacharia was 18. Soon afterwards his father died of a heart attack. The family was reduced to poverty. Zacharia and his 16-year-old brother Omar got embroiled with criminals when they tried to get money for the family. Omar was shot dead from a passing car when Zacharia was in his company. Following that, Zacharia started abusing drugs. Afterwards, Zacharia's oldest brother Karim managed to rehabilitate the garage. He refused to employ Zacharia in the garage. He and the rest of the family blamed Zacharia for having dragged Omar into crime and failed to protect him. Since then Zacharia had been excommunicated by his family of origin, but his mother and his grandmother on her side continued supporting him secretly, emotionally and financially. They helped him rehabilitate. He stopped abusing drugs and could support himself by odd jobs.

Zacharia met Rodica, a foreign worker from Romania, in a local supermarket. She got married to him but could not speak Arabic and was rejected by her neighbors. Her family in Romania objected to her marriage with a Muslim man and severed all ties with her. Even before her pregnancy she fell into depression and tried to commit suicide with pills. After Bassel was born she suffered from postpartum depression and couldn't take care of him. She committed suicide when Bassel was six-months-old. The circumstances of her death were kept secret from Bassel, but he knew. Following her death, Zacharia began to use drugs again, on and off.

Zacharia's family of origin refused to have any contact with Bassel, on the pretext of his being the son of Zacharia and a Christian foreigner they considered to be "crazy". It was not easy for Zacharia's mother and grandmother to be in touch with Bassel, because they were exposed to the intrusive eyes of the family and the neighbors.

Half a year after Rodica's death, Zacharia married Yasmina, a Muslim Arab woman from an Arab village. People gossiped about her that she had been compelled to leave her community because of her unacceptable behavior. She used to dress in modern attire without a head cover. She had attended a seminar for teachers. She liked to read and do crafts, and had ambitions, but gave it all up when she got married to Zacharia. She was bitter and discontented, both because of her frustrated aspirations and because she felt that Zacharia still missed his deceased wife, and wanted her, Yasmina, only as a housewife and as caregiver for Bassel.

Yasmina got pregnant only after years of fertility treatments, when Bassel approached the age of eight.

Bassel was placed in a nursery school when he was three-years-old. Right from the very beginning he was socially rejected, failing to fit into group activities or understand social situations. When the nursery school teachers complained about his bullying, Zacharia was trying to teach him a lesson by beating him up. But then he would regret it and keep away from him.

Bassel was very interested in cars. He knew all the car brands. He used to play with toy cars. Every now and again he would go to his uncle's garage and watch it from the outside. Once he was courageous and entered the garage. His uncle drove him out.

A classified list of publications

Multi-systemic diagnosis and therapy

Ariel, S. (2002). *Children's imaginative play: A visit to Wonderland.* Westport, CT: Praeger.
Ariel, S. (2018). *Multi-dimensional therapy with families, children and adults: The Diamond Model.* London, UK: Routledge.

Brooks-Harris, J.E. (2007). *Integrative multi-theoretical psychotherapy.* Boston, MA: Cengage Learning.

Erskine, R.G. (2015). *Relational patterns, therapeutic presence: Concepts and practice of integrative psychotherapy.* London, UK: Routledge.

Finale, L. (2015). *Relational integrative psychotherapy: Engaging process and theory in practice.* Hoboken, NJ: Wiley-Blackwell.

Chapter 14

Planning a therapeutic strategy

The diagnostic evaluation serves as a basis for designing an overall strategy, or a number of alternative strategies, for the therapy. A strategy determines the therapeutic goals and the main ways for reaching them. They attempt to predict obstacles on the ways of reaching the goals and offer ways of removing or overcoming them.

In designing strategies, it is important to base every decision on explicit considerations, which take into account the information collected in the evaluation phase. A strategy is just a general treatment plan. It should not be adhered to rigidly during the therapy. It will be modified flexibly, adapted to new data encountered in the various stages of therapy.

The questions that should be asked when a strategy is designed are:

(a) What are the specific targets of change?

In the Diamond Model the main targets of change are the bugs in the various information-processing programs. The therapy should concentrate primarily on removing or weakening such bugs. Bugs prevent the homeostasis-maintaining mechanisms from functioning properly. Removing or weakening the bugs can restore the systems' ability to mobilize corrective, balance-maintaining feedback. It will be recalled also that bugs are kinds of defenses, energized by over-heated emotions. A preliminary for removing or weakening the bugs is therefore restoring the balance of unbalanced emotions that are associated with emotives to which the bugs are related.

Bugs are also influenced by the clients' developmental profiles

In designing the strategy, one has to decide first which of the bugs to concentrate on.

(b) What kinds of difficulties can one expect to encounter on the way of trying to restore emotion-balance and remove the bugs?

The difficulties can come from various origins: Lack of motivation or resistance to change, lack of strengths or skills required, failure of the therapeutic alliance, low level of development in programs and dimensions relevant to the therapy, etc. It is necessary therefore, in the stage of planning strategies, to assess in advance factors that can contribute to the therapy's success vs. factors that can adversely affect the therapy. Among such factors are, for instance, the nature and strength of motivation for therapy of each of the participants, sources and motives of resistance, strengths and weaknesses of the clients, cultural and personality traits that can assist or hamper the prospects of success.

One should also be alert to possible adverse effect that can be caused by careless therapeutic moves.

(c) What is the order of priorities in choosing intervention foci?

The main consideration is efficiency. One should concentrate first on trying to intervene in foci that are expected to get the best results with the least resistance and investment of time and efforts. A relevant metaphor is the domino effect. One should prefer to achieve changes that will lead spontaneously to other changes in the desired directions. One should also try to predict possible adverse effects that can be caused by the intervention.

When designing a strategy, it is advisable to make first a list of the programs of the participants in the case, and the bugs found in these programs. One should distinguish between programs that are still relevant on the one hand, and programs that belong to the history of the case but are not relevant anymore to its current state.

Interdisciplinary seminar

Shlomo: Let's design a strategy for Gad's case (Case 13.1). What are the treatment goals? What do we want to achieve?

Anna: First, we want to help Gad. That was the purpose of the referral. I don't know, I feel that Esther and Benny need help too. Not only as a means of helping Gad but as an end in itself. Everyone in this family suffers.

Shlomo: This is obvious. Although this was not defined as the purpose of referral, it is impossible to treat Gad's difficulties as unrelated to the difficulties of the entire family. In summarizing the diagnostic assessment, we referred to parts of the developmental profiles of the family members, their emotives and the bugs in their proximity and control plans. We have seen that these three types of entities feed each other. In planning the strategy, we must choose the elements of development, the unbalanced emotives and the bugs to which we will direct most of our therapeutic efforts. We will give priority to change purposes which, if achieved, would be followed by other spontaneous changes. But at the same time, we will take into account possible obstacles to achieving the desired changes and even possible negative consequences of our interventions.

The frameworks of the therapy – individual, family, group, community or combinations of frameworks, as well as the therapeutic methods and techniques employed, will be chosen on the basis of these strategic considerations.

Anna: I don't know where to start, but I think it is important that Gad gets medical treatment and rehabilitation for his objective difficulties. Drug therapy for his metabolic dysfunction along with appropriate diets, medication along with techniques to improve attention and concentration, activities to improve motor skills. I don't know which treatments exist for sensory over-sensitivity.

Shlomo: All these can be improved by play therapy techniques. Esther doesn't seem to have done anything with Odeda's diagnosis, nor have the school provided any treatment.

Ethan: Not at all surprising. We said that Esther's control goals with respect to Gad were to mold him in the shape of her own ideal self and to protect him from external influences. She also denied his difficulties, interpreted them as just superficial external expressions.

Shlomo: As I said, we must take obstacles such as resistance into consideration.

Daniel: We said that these bugs were energized by projecting on Gad her fear of not being appreciated and effaced as a person. To remove these bugs, a way should be found to balance these emotive-related emotions.

Lailah: And also help her to become aware of the fact that she projects on Gad her own difficulties with herself. Remove the horse blinders.

Ethan: It seems that many problems would be solved if the bugs in Esther's proximity and control plans with respect to Gad, Benny, her parents, the school or any other body were weakened or removed. This could be achieved if her emotive-related emotions were balanced and her empathy capacity developed. Then she wouldn't deny Gad's objective difficulties and the need to let professionals other than you and Odeda provide treatment. She would perhaps see her mother's involvement in raising and educating him in a positive light and would start a dialogue with her. Maybe she would even allow her father to serve as a grandfather, considering the possibility that as a grandfather to a male grandson he might be much softer than as a father to a daughter. She would see Benny's assets and the need to empower him and let him have a more central and dominant place as husband and father, despite his physical disability. I would give the task of helping her get rid of her bugs the highest priority, because the success of this move could open the way for further changes in the desired direction.

Lailah: We talked about obstacles? Resistance? She was highly invested in her emotives, in her difficulty to summon empathy and in her bugs, because all these had very deep roots in her childhood. I would perhaps start with an individual therapy with her, let her have a place of her own and delve deeper. In one-to-one conversation with a lot of empathy and emotional support, it might be possible to help her recognize Gad's objective difficulties and persuade her to let the right professionals provide treatment.

Anna: Maybe it would be a good idea to offer Benny a parallel individual therapy, to empower him and help him discover his own strengths and abilities, Odeda with Esther and Shlomo with Benny. I would encourage Benny to seek professional rehabilitation, re-training. After that I would do individual play therapy with Gad.

This could serve various purposes. He could be himself, without pressure to act against his will and his limited abilities. He will be treated with respect, to reduce his fear of being the object of derision and mockery. The right play-therapeutic techniques can help him improve his motor skills. Only after the emotional difficulties of each of the three will be worked through in individual therapy will there be a higher chance of success of family play therapy aimed at weakening the bugs in the mutual proximity-control relationships between the family members.

Daniel: I think Esther's parents should participate in the family play therapy, after Esther's being prepared to accept them. Consulting the school is also needed. The school staff can help Gad strengthen his self-confidence and integrate into society. For example, he would be encouraged to introduce his knowledge of vehicles to his class mates.

Ethan: Afterwards I would have Gad participate in group play therapy to help him understand his own share in his social isolation, to correctly interpret his peers' reactions to him, and to explore his possible contributions to society.

Anna: Is that what you meant by the concept of strategy?

Shlomo: Yes, at this point there is no need to go into more detail.

Anna: It would be a very complex therapy, with multiple ingredients.

Shlomo: As I see it, each case is multi-systemic and therefore the therapy is also complex and multi-dimensional. If we do not take into account all the relevant elements, the therapy is in danger of failing and can even be harmful. Suppose for instance that Esther yield to pressures to provide Gad with rehabilitative treatments that would expose his limitations but would also show that his strengths and areas of interest lie very far from the areas that she was trying to educate and shape him on. Unless Esther is prepared to accept this through individual and family therapy, she may undermine Gad's achievements, intensify the pressure on him and cause a regression.

We can continue to develop ideas about strategy, but it seems to me that the basic principles are understood.

Summary of chapter 14

The multi-systemic diagnostic evaluation serves as a basis for designing an overall strategy, or a number of alternative strategies, for the therapy. A strategy determines the therapeutic goals and the main ways for reaching them. It attempts to predict obstacles on the ways of reaching the goals and offer ways of removing or overcoming them. A strategy should not be adhered to rigidly during the therapy. A question that should be asked when a strategy is designed is: What are the specific targets of change? The main targets are bugs in the various relevant programs. Removing or weakening the bugs can restore the systems' ability to mobilize corrective, balance-maintaining feedback. Bugs are energized by overheated emotions. A preliminary for removing or weakening the bugs is therefore restoring the balance of unbalanced emotions that are associated with emotives to which the bugs are related. Bugs are also influenced by the clients' developmental profiles. In designing the strategy, one has to decide first which of the bugs to concentrate on. Priority will be given to creating a domino effect, that is, removing bugs that, if removed, will lead to more and more spontaneous changes in the desired direction. Another consideration would be predicting the kinds of difficulties one can expect to encounter on the way of trying to restore emotion-balance and remove the bugs. The difficulties can come from various origins. In the stage of planning strategies, it is necessary to assess in advance factors that can contribute to the therapy's success vs. factors that can adversely affect the therapy.

> **Assignments**
>
> Propose two alternative strategies for the case of Bassel (Case 13.2) – targets of change, priorities and possible obstacles. Compare the two strategies and decide which of them is better. Justify your choice.

A classified list of publications

Multi-dimensional therapeutic strategies

Ariel, S. (2018). *Multi-dimensional therapy with families, children and adults: The Diamond Model*. London, UK: Routledge.

Pinsof, W.M. and Breunlin, D. (2017). *Integrative systemic therapy: Metaframeworks for problem solving with individual, couples and families*. Washington, DC: American Psychological Association.

Wagner, W.G. (2002). *Counseling, psychology and children: A multi-dimensional approach to interventions*. Upper Saddle River, NJ: Prentice Hall.

Part 5

How to do it?

Chapter 15
Conducting a play-therapeutic session

The role of the play therapist

In this genre of therapy, the therapist is an active participant in the spontaneous play of the individual child, the family or the group. The therapeutic goals are achieved by three kinds of play moves: *Main moves*, in which the emotion-balancing techniques and the bug-busters are subtly activated; *preparatory moves*, preparing the ground for the main moves; and *auxiliary moves*, controlling unwanted side effects of preparatory or main moves. Preparatory and auxiliary moves have various functions such as joining, influencing the course of the play, supporting, focusing attention and emphasizing, commenting, reflecting and interpreting. These are achieved by playful techniques, belonging to a given repertoire or made up by the therapist. Here is a sample of such techniques:

Mimicking the clients' play

Therapeutic functions:

Joining. When children want to join a play activity, they simply imitate the play of children they want to play with. The therapist can do the same.
Reflecting, commenting. By imitating aspects of the clients' play behavior, such as an accusing finger pointed by a mother at her daughter, the therapist reflects those aspects and comments on them.

Pacing

Therapeutic functions: Channeling play behavior to specific routes, which prepare the ground for the main moves.

After the therapist mimics the play of a client, she gradually modifies her own play, until the clients begin to imitate her play. For example, a child is playing as if he is a very noisy elephant. The therapist is mimicking his play, pretending to be another noisy elephant. But then the therapist is gradually lowering her voice, until the child has become a quiet elephant.

Focusing

Therapeutic functions: Stressing aspects of the play behavior, by sound and lighting effects or by verbal and non-verbal comments; interpreting.

In a family play therapy session, a girl wanted her mother to play with her at leisure. The mother was impatient, as if hurrying to finish the game and move on to something else. The therapist reacted by whistling the song "I'm late, I'm late for a very important date", from Disney's adaptation of *Alice in Wonderland*.

Explicating

Therapeutic functions: Making hidden entities explicit, by verbalizing them or acting them out non-verbally; emphasizing important features; interpreting.

A family staged "a bank robbery" make-believe game. To explicate the family members' covert messages, the therapist assumed the role of a TV reporter at the end of the scene. She interviewed "the bank manager", "the police officer", "the witness" and "the robber" about their motives for acting as they did and about their feelings.

The double

Therapeutic functions: The therapist, directly or through a doll, speaks for a client who refuses to participate in the play activity or is unable to express his hidden feelings and thoughts.

In a family play therapy, a mother, speaking through a doll, poured a torrent of accusations on her son, who remained silent. His mother accused him of treating her with disrespect because he didn't answer her. The therapist took hold of a doll which was identical to the son's and said, "I can't talk. I'm too afraid to talk."

Providing stimuli

Therapeutic functions: Encouraging certain kinds of activities or changing the course of an activity.

To encourage a girl to express her jealousy of her newly born brother, the therapist placed near her a baby doll, a baby cradle and other baby things.

Illusion of alternatives

Therapeutic functions: The therapist suggests two alternative play ideas. The more attractive alternative is the one he wants the client to choose. This enables the therapist to join the clients' play or influence its course.

A therapist who wanted to encourage a timid little boy to express his strong side in play asked the boy: "Do you prefer being Mickey Mouse of Mighty Mouse?"

Obedient actor

Therapeutic functions: The therapist asks clients for permission to join their play and lets them choose her role in it. Once inside, she is free to make her own choices. This enables the therapist to become an equal play partner.

Willy-nilly

Therapeutic functions: The therapist performs a play act that engages the client in a complementary play act. In this way, the therapist manages to involve the child in play in accordance with the therapist's aims.

A therapist who wanted to cast a boy in the role of a hunter said to him, "I am the rabbit. Hunter, please don't' shoot me!"

Some of these techniques have been observed in children's spontaneous play. Others have been borrowed from Milton Erickson and other strategic therapists, e.g. Erickson and Rossi, 1980; Madanes, 1991.

Interdisciplinary seminar

Anna: Can the same types of moves be made in individual play therapy, family play therapy and group play therapy?

Shlomo: Yes. In the kind of play therapy that's informed by the Diamond Model, individual play therapy is, in a way, a dyadic group play therapy with a therapist and a client. Family play therapy may also be considered a subtype of group play therapy. This, I believe, will become clearer once I'll have introduced you to some vignettes from individual, family and group play therapy with Gad and his family (Case 13.1).

Individual play therapy

Session 15.1 Gad

Gad is sitting with his back to me. His toy truck is again inside a walled enclosure. Other toy trucks are scattered around the room. Gad takes his toy truck out of the enclosure. He makes it run fast, noisily and collide with other trucks. After he hits a truck, he throws it away.

I let him do it without intervening. I wonder how I can enter his play. After all, he refuses to let anyone into his play world. I take a toy helicopter, lift it in the air with my right arm, fly it around the area where Gad is playing and make a thrumming helicopter sound. I hold a toy microphone in my left hand and talk into it, "Police helicopter traffic control! Multiple road accident near the house that's surrounded by a double wall. Trucks damaged. No casualties seen so far." Gad doesn't ignore me. He is looking at the helicopter, intrigued.

Anna: His play reminds me of the play with his parents. Maybe he repeats more or less the same play over and over again as a means of achieving emotion- balance – anger at the children he sees as hostile, anger at his father. The tossing of the trucks reminds me of the pile of broken cars that included his father's car. One of his emotives is anger at his father's impotence and passivity.

Lailah: I think the cop on the helicopter gave Gad a message that he is not necessarily a victim, that he is aggressive and can cause harm. I don't know if you're meant to deliver such a message, but it seems to me that it can somewhat weaken the bugs, horse blinders and non-sense.

Ethan: I understand that the problem you were trying to solve was how to get Gad to accept you as his play partner. You didn't invade his territory and chose a suitable role, which naturally fits into the content of his play. You remained in a position of observer and reflector. It seems to me that out of the list of joining techniques, you chose focusing, explicating and willy-nilly. Although Gad did not invite you to play with him, you did succeed in arousing his curiosity and interest. He did not ignore you as he usually does.

Shlomo: Interesting observations. Let's continue.

Session 15.1 (2) Gad, contd.

I am putting on a blue hat and get various toy tools. I start "fixing" the trucks Gad threw. Gad is watching me silently. With my right hand, I take the police helicopter and make it descend from the air to the floor. I change the blue hat with a toy helmet and talk in a cop's voice, "Who are you and what are you doing here?" I put on the blue hat again and say, "I am a mechanic. I'm fixing these damaged trucks." I continue to play both roles.

Cop: Did you see what happened?

Mechanic: The blue truck over there lost control of the steering wheel, collided with these trucks forcefully. They were pushed to all sides and were damaged.

Cop: Were there people in the damaged trucks? Are there causalities?

Mechanic: No. The trucks were empty. They were here in the truck depot.

Cop: Did the driver hit the truck on purpose?

Mechanic: No, no. He lost control of the steering wheel.

At this point, Gad says indignantly, "No! I did it on purpose!"

I say, "Let's play as if he pretended that he didn't do it on purpose. He did it on purpose because he imagined the trucks were going to hit him, but let's play as if he didn't imagine such a thing. The mechanic didn't want him to get into trouble with the police."

Gad (whispering), "He didn't do it."

Cop: OK.

I make the helicopter go away.

Anna: At first I thought "Is this play therapy? Shlomo did all the play!", but then I understood that what you did were what you call preparatory moves. You gradually got Gad first interested in your play and then begin taking part in it, however small.

Lailah: I liked it that you played two make-believe roles. The play allowed you a great deal of flexibility.

Ethan: Your choice of playing the role of a mechanic was right in my opinion. First of all, it adapted itself to the situation: You damaged the trucks and I repaired the damage. If I'm not mistaken, it was also an indirect message to Gad, "I am here to help, to fix things." Perhaps even a control goal, " I will protect you from yourself, from your aggression, without being critical."

Daniel: You sent Gad a message that his aggression was not intentional, but rather a result of losing control of the steering wheel. This may have been an indirect message about his violence towards children in school. It is interesting that he insisted that his aggression was intentional.

Lailah: Perhaps because it made him look weak and out of control, not as someone who knows how to defend himself and hurt those who hurt him.

Ethan: You said, "Let's play as if he pretended that he didn't do it on purpose. The mechanic didn't want him to get into trouble with the police." By saying this you emphasized that this was make-believe play, and you managed to draw him into the play. The use of the third person and the past tense to indicate imagined time, as well as the separation between the character and the person playing this character (basic duality) and make-believe within make-believe ("play as if you pretended"), allowed Gad to distance himself from his own aggression without giving up, and be aware of its implications (lifting horse blinders). You also said, "He did it on purpose because he imagined the trucks were going to hit him, but let's play as if he didn't imagine such a thing." If I understand correctly, by that move you referred to the fact that he attacks friends even if they approach him with good intentions. You hinted that he sometimes imagines their bad intentions. You used the bug-buster owning and alienation to instill in him the idea that his attribution may have been wrong, while allowing him to keep this attribution without giving it up.

Shlomo: Well done! Exact use of the concepts of analysis you have learned.

Anna: Was this a main move or a preparatory move?

Shlomo: Main move. Many main moves can be made during the therapy.

Session 15.1 (3) Gad, contd.

Shlomo: Let's pretend the mechanic couldn't fix the trucks. I can't! I give up!

Gad: They can't be fixed. They are ruined.

Shlomo: I am sure they can be fixed. I am going to try again. First, I'll get rid of these flat tires. This truck will run better without tires.

Gad (makes a disdainful face): It won't go without tires.

Shlomo (surprised): Really? OK, we don't need its damaged engine. A horse can be harnessed to it and it will go easily. And it will not need gas.

Gad: That's stupid.

Shlomo: Let's play as if he was a stupid mechanic and the other guy was the best mechanic in the world. I know you are an excellent mechanic. Will you accept me as an apprentice? Let's pretend he agreed. Teach me how to fix this truck.

Gad: It needs a new engine. All its parts should be replaced. It will not pay-off fixing it.

Shlomo: All right, just teach me how to fix it right. This truck will only be used to demonstrate repairs.

Gad: First you need to know all the external and internal parts of vehicles.

Shlomo: Can you teach me?

Gad: Yes.

Shlomo: Let's pretend now is after two years, and the stupid mechanic learned from the best mechanic in the world all one needs to know to fix a truck.

I stack all the trucks into a pile and say, "This was a dump of scrap trucks. The stupid mechanic started a business of renovating old trucks. He would take trucks from the pile, renovate them and sell them to collectors.

"Sir, are you a collector?" Let's pretend he said, "yes". "Are you interested in a renovated truck?"

Gad: Yes.

Shlomo: I have an offer for you at a bargain price. Do you see this truck?

I show Gad a large, heavy toy truck which looks very massive and strong but stained with ugly patches, with scratches and cracks all over, not very attractive.

Shlomo: I'm telling you that even if it doesn't look very impressive, it is a truck with a turbocharger with a million-horsepower engine, with the best performance in the world. It is the fastest, immune to accidents and can climb cliffs and fly. You will be proud to have such a wonderful truck and to be the one who drives it.

Gad: How much?

Shlomo: Only a million dollars. It's nothing.

Gad makes a gesture as if he is giving me money. He takes the truck and begins to drive it fast across the room, making it climb the walls and fly. But suddenly he knocks it down on the floor and says, "It stopped working, it's worthless. You cheated me. Take it back and give me my money!"

Shlomo: It's just the battery. You made it work hard for a whole year and the battery became exhausted. Let me replace it.

I am pretending to replace the battery. Gad resumes his driving the truck very fast in all directions. But after a while, he places the truck on the floor, lay on his back on the floor and doesn't move. Then he gets up, takes the blue truck with which he hit the trucks before, puts it inside the construction with the double walls and closes the external wall with play blocks.

I surround the blocks constructions with the trucks that Gad had hit before and say, "Let's pretend the enemy trucks were besieging the building with the walls."

I am handing Gad over the big, "ugly" turbo truck I had given him before and say, "The stupid assistant suggested that this powerful truck should be with the blue truck inside the wall. The blue truck needs reinforcement."

Gad takes the "ugly" turbo truck and throws it away. Then I am getting a big transparent plastic bag and say, "I'm your assistant. The walls are not strong enough to withstand an attack from all sides and certainly not an attack from the air. This is a transparent dome, made of completely impenetrable material. It can provide you with full protection from all directions, including from above. You don't need the bricks walls. They can be easily destroyed. This transparent dome has another advantage, you can have a full view of what's going on outside and be prepared to defend your truck."

Gad takes the transparent plastic bag and covers with it the whole construction with the truck inside.

I'm saying, "Now you don't need the walls. They are useless, and they disturb your view."

Gad ignores me.

Anna: Again, it was you who did most of the playing. It was mainly your play, not his, although you focused on his favorite theme, vehicles. Wouldn't it be more like play therapy if you let Gad initiate his own play and you would intervene only in some suitable junctions?

Shlomo: Case-by-case. I would be less directive with clients who initiate their own original, evolving play and allow the therapist to join their play. Gad played in a stereotypical and repetitive manner, doing the same acts again and again and not letting me or anyone else play with him. My goal was to encourage him to accept me as a playmate, help him develop and enrich his play in therapeutically relevant ways. As you saw, he gradually accepted me as a partner and brought some of his own contents. Later, he initiated more and more play moves of his own. Then I retreated and took a less directive role.

Lailah: I like it that you took a one-down position, pretending to be a dumb mechanic, making absurd and funny suggestions, like harnessing the damaged truck to a horse. Then you asked Gad to be his apprentice – control role and plan, letting Gad control you. You gave Gad, indirectly, through the make-believe play, two important messages: First, no total loss, the truck can be fixed by a competent mechanic. Second, you are such a competent mechanic. You can fix the truck and teach me how to be a good mechanic. I think these messages allude, through the basic duality of play, both to Gad's seeing his father as a kind of total loss, and to Gad seeing himself as damaged and incompetent. Your interventions were designed, the way I see it, to give him hope, to help him believe that things and people can be improved, to emphasize his own assets and his possible positive contributions to other people.

Daniel: When you said "Now it's after two years and the stupid mechanic learned how to fix a truck", you made use of the identication of the play time with future imaginary time. I thought this was a message to Gad that he can look ahead for improvement. The pile of scrap trucks was taken of course from Gad's own play (Observation 13.1). He said that his father was, as it were, an irreparably damaged truck on this pile. You insisted that he can be renovated, rehabilitated.

Ethan: When you sold him a large, bulky, ugly renovated truck, of which the unimpressive exterior does not attest to its wonderful interior, I thought you referred indirectly to his poor self-image. You conveyed him the message that despite his physical limitations, he had many strengths, an unrealized potential. You said he should be proud of this truck. It seems that you alluded to his emotive of shame for having the limitations he had.

Anna: He was influenced by your suggestive statements and did with the truck acrobatic tricks like in the play you described to us (Observation 13.1), but suddenly he dropped the truck on the floor, said it was worthless and accused you of cheating him. It seems that he wasn't sure he could trust you and believe in your encouraging messages. It seems to me that this was also a manifestation of the mechanism of fluctuations. Going back to the peak of his emotive of feeling incompetent. But he was stuck there, could not distance himself again from the core of his emotive to its less depressive, more euphoric periphery. He needed your help as a play therapist to use this emotion-balancing technique, so you came up with the replacing the battery idea. It did work for a while, but afterwards he stopped, took a rest for a while and got his blue truck, his own original choice, into the safe, walled structure. He rejected your "ugly" turbo truck. Again, the emotion-balancing of play. Then you came up with the idea of the siege and the transparent plastic bag, a playful emotion-balancing move. He partly co-operated, covered the construction with the plastic bag, but to be on the safe side kept the play blocks walls.

Ethan: You used the bug-buster arbitrariness of the dignified to bust the bugs horse blinders and fifth wheel. The plastic bag idea was an arbitrary signifier, an easily penetrable and seen through material, for the signified content impenetrable dome. This was a playful way of conveying the message that hiding, isolating himself and surrounding himself with a wall is not necessary and irrelevant to his current life situation.

Family play therapy

Shlomo: Excellent analyses. Let's inspect some vignettes from play therapy with Gad's family. The family sessions began after a period of individual meetings with Gad, when our therapeutic relationship had been established and Gad was willing and ready to share the treatment with his parents.

Anna: It seems that the therapy was not conducted according to the strategy we proposed. For example, the family therapy did not take place after individual therapy with each of the parents.

Shlomo: The actual therapy had been conducted way before we worked out the strategy. Don't forget that our purpose here is not to present a full description of the case, but just to illustrate some of the concepts and methods we have learned.

Session 15.2 Gad, Benny and Esther

Gad scatters trucks and cars across the room. He drives his blue truck very fast, deliberately targeting and colliding with trucks and other cars.

Benny is sitting in the corner of the room, doing nothing.

Esther puts on a police hat. She is holding a toy steering wheel, as if driving a traffic police car. She is holding a play block. She approaches Gad, talking into the block as if it is a police radio mic, "Highway patrol! Pull over!"

Gad ignores her. She looks at me, helpless. I'm telling her, "Let's pretend the cop called traffic police headquarters."

I'm putting on a police hat and wear a toy radio device with earphones and a mic.

She is talking to the block, "Headquarters, a driver here runs wild on the road, hits vehicles and refuses my call to pull over."

I'm saying, "Give me your location. I'll send in reinforcement."

I am mumbling, as if to myself, "We have a problem of manpower. We recruited retired cops, the best, senior officers who know how to work with their heads."

I am approaching Benny, saying, "Officer, we have a situation in Highway 500. A driver rages on the road, hits vehicles, ignores the calls to pull over. Take your cops there and deal with the problem."

Benny smiles with embarrassment.

I'm telling him, "Lets make-believe that now is before he retired, when he was the best."

Benny is asking, "What should I do?"

Shlomo: "Now you are not you, you are a high officer who knows what to do."

Benny: "OK." He is getting up, limping toward Gad and says, "All police cars! Put a road block and stop this truck and arrest the driver."

He is giggling, laying his hand on Gad's shoulder. Gad stands up. They face each other.

Esther is saying, "You should arrest him!"

Benny says, "No need to. He is not going to do it again."

Esther: He needs to participate in a defensive driving skills course. I teach such courses.

Shlomo: Yes, her's is the best defensive driving skills school in the whole country. It has won numerous awards and has provided generations of good drivers. But first he will have to stand trial and be punished for traffic violations and damages caused to vehicles. He is a minor. Where are his parents?

Gad points to his parents and says "here".

I say: Are these your parents?

He says: Yes.

I tell Esther: No. If he is your son, he will not be allowed to take a defensive driving skills course at your school. During the difficult period he is going to go through, what he will need is a lot of love and emotional support from his parents. A preventive driving skills course he will take in another school.

Let's play as if the daddy and mommy, who were themselves cops, escorted the offending driver to the police station for investigation. I'll be the investigating policeman. On the way to the station they encourage the minor driver, calm him down and tell him how much they love him. But if he doesn't let them touch him or talk to him, they pretend they do not care, and they play as if they are indifferent.

Benny and Esther put their hands on Gad's shoulders and whisper encouraging words to him. As expected, he removes their hands. They take their hands off his shoulders and pretend to be indifferent. He looks at them puzzled.

Anna: I see that at the beginning Gad's play repeated itself, despite the previous individual sessions, and also that Benny was still sitting passively on the side, but Esther began to initiate her own make-believe play, without you having to encourage her. Playing highway patrol was a part of her plan to reach her control goal with respect to Gad. But he ignored her.

Lailah: Esther looked at you helpless and at this point you joined the play in a supportive and superior role as an officer in HQ.

Ethan: It seems that these were preparatory moves toward the main moves, designed to boost Benny's self-concept and get him involved in the play in a dominant role. You said, "We recruited retired cops, the best, senior officers who know how to work with their heads." By saying this you challenged his self-concept as "retired" and communicated to him the message, "Even if you are physically incapacitated, you can still use your brain." Again, you used distancing, third person and past tense, to make it easier for him to overcome his inhibition, by reinforcing the owning and alienation of the play.

Daniel: You said, "Lets make-believe that now is before he retired, when he was the best." You used the identication of the present time with the past time, when Benny was better. You also said, "Now you are not you, you are a high officer who knows what to do." I think you applied the basic duality and owning and alienation to bust his horse blinders and non-sense concerning his capacities and the role he can play as a parent.

Lailah: This move was effective. Gad didn't resist. He stood up and faced Benny.

Anna: For Esther it won't be easy to accept Benny as a dominant parental figure. She activated her control plan by first telling Benny, "You should arrest him" and then by offering herself as a defensive-driving-skills teacher for Gad, trying to reestablish her role as Gad's sole educator and teacher. You told her, "Her's is the best defensive-driving-skills school. It provided generations of good drivers." The message was, "You are not invisible, you are an excellent parent, educator and teacher." But you conveyed the message that what Gad needs from her (and from Benny) is love, warmth and support, not teaching. The bug buster of possible worlds was activated when they took your idea and escorted Gad with supporting words. Gad wasn't used to such an attitude on their part, so he was ambivalent, flip-flop.

Shlomo: Excellent!

Group play therapy

I'd like now to move on to the subject of peer-group play therapy.

A child is invited to participate only if ready, usually following individual and family sessions. Preparedness refers to the question of whether the child is ripe for an advanced group activity in terms of his or her level of development and emotional state. Another consideration is the question whether he or she is likely to sabotage the group activity due to uncontrolled behavior.

My kind of group play therapy is unstructured. The session begins with a brief structured activity, a game, rhythmical drumming, movement exercises or the like. The participants are asked to remind themselves the basic rules of conduct in the room, e.g. no violence (make-believe violence is not forbidden), not to insult or harass one another, no damage to property, security precautions (e.g. not to touch the electricity socket, not to kick a ball at a lamp), not to leave the room without permission, etc. Afterwards, the children play freely, not necessarily together. The therapist joins the play by various preparatory moves. The main moves (accompanied by auxiliary moves when necessary), like in individual or family play therapy, can be aimed at emotive-related emotion-balancing, busting bugs in proximity-control plans and enhancing development. The moves are informed by the therapist's knowledge of the difficulties of each participant, as well as by what's going on in the children' play. If the play gets out of control, deteriorates into frenzy, unruly behavior or violence, the therapist stops the play and reverts to a structured, calming down activity, until the children are ready to resume free play.

The session ends with a short-structured activity. The therapist summarizes the session, points out what has been achieved and praises each of the participants for his or her accomplishments. The summary can be done in a playful way, e.g. through puppets.

In the meeting in which we discussed the emotion-balancing functions of make-believe play, I told you about a strong, vigorous, dominant eight-year-old boy, Rex, who in a group play therapy suddenly began playing as if he was seriously ill and died. I learned from his mother that his father was diagnosed with leukemia. (Session 11.1). Gad participated in this group, which consisted of three boys and two girls, all around the age of eight. The other members of the group, apart from Rex and Gad, were a timid boy named Yuri, an active, dominant girl named Sophia and a shy girl named Zoe.

Session 15.3 Group play therapy with Gad

Gad is sitting in the corner of the room, his back turned to the others, moving a toy truck to-and-fro.

Zoe is sitting on a chair, just observing the others.

Yuri is disguised as a witch.

Rex kicks a spongy ball, with power, toward Sophia. She kicks the ball back to him.

Rex kicks the ball toward Yuri. The latter is running, climbing on a chair. He declares, "I am the witch! I am the queen of the world."

Rex is walking toward him. Yuri recoils. Rex is touching his leg. Yuri whines, "No!"

Rex is kicking the ball toward Zoe. The latter smiles uneasily and doesn't respond.

When Rex is standing with his back toward Yuri, the latter is running toward Rex, blows air in the back of his neck and is running back fast to his chair, climbing on it.

Rex is approaching Gad, standing behind him. Gad ignores him. Rex bounces the ball lightly on Gad's back. Gad is saying, "Stop it!" angrily. Rex continues. Gad is getting up, standing in front of Rex with a menacing pose.

I am approaching Rex, saying, "Ronaldo, you forgot I am the coach? Do you want to add him to the team as a goal keeper or do you think he is a fan and would be happy to have your attention?"

Rex says, "Join him to the team as a goalkeeper."

I say, "Too soon. True, he is a brilliant future soccer player but I'm not sure he wants to devote himself to soccer, and if he does, he will need a long period of training before he is fit to join the team. But meanwhile he can be our driver, who drives us to games."

Gad is looking at me, hesitating, and then goes back to his truck.

Rex says, "Let's play as if the coach was ill and couldn't train him, but no one knew he was ill."

I am sitting down on an armchair, reclining backwards. I am covering myself with a blanket and sigh, "Oh, I feel bad, I'm sick, I can't train the team."

Sophia is putting on a nurse cap and says, "I am the nurse, I'll cure him." (She did the same when Rex had pretended to be ill in the play described in Observation 11.1.)

Yuri, still standing on the chair, is saying, "The witch cured him by her magic healing power."

Shlomo: (Sighs) Her healing magic power doesn't work from afar. She has to fly close to the ill or injured person for it to work. I know this from the games of our soccer team. When a player was lying on the grass wounded, she would fly to him, invisible, heal him, and he could get up and continue playing.

Yuri is getting off the chair. He approaches me, looking at Rex anxiously. He is bringing his palm close above me, saying, "Heal now! Heal now!"

I rise, emit a sigh of relief and say, "I feel much better!"

I approach Zoe and say, "In our next soccer game you won't be sitting on the bench. You'll be in the game with us."

Zoe is not responding. I'm saying, "Do you want to play with us next time?"

"Let's pretend she didn't know," says Zoe.

Rex is calling out, alarmed, "Oh no! Our coach is ill again!"

I am sitting down on the armchair, reclined back. I am sighing. I whisper, "I feel much worse, like."

Sophia is putting on again the nurse cap and coming toward me. She is holding a plastic bottle. She is saying, "Drink this medicine."

Yuri is running toward me. He is bringing his palm close above me, saying, "Heal now! Heal now!"

Rex: It won't work! He's going to die!

Shlomo: Call an ambulance, please! Let's pretend they took him to the hospital and he got better. Let's play as if Gad was the ambulance driver and he took him to the hospital.

Gad is taking a big toy ambulance, driving it fast toward me.

Shlomo: Lets play as if all of you help the coach get into the ambulance and stay with him inside it on the way to the hospital, in case he needs help.

Zoe is getting up from her chair. She is mumbling something into a toy smartphone. She is saying, "I am calling the hospital and telling them to prepare a bed for him."

Lailah: This is very different from the kind of group therapy I learned, in which the participants sit together and go through a conjoint dynamic group process.

Daniel: In what ways is it different?

Lailah: It's less focused. It is also hard for me to see a linear process of group development.

Shlomo: It is not that different. Although the children don't sit together and each of them is busy doing his own thing, one can easily notice the proximity-control goals and plans the children have with respect to each other. I described only a short section of the group play, but that group also underwent a gradual process of change in their proximity-control relationships, alongside with emotion-balancing processes around the children's emotives and a great deal of learning and development on the interpersonal level.

Anna: I see that despite the individual and family therapy it was not easy at all to help Gad out of his entrenching himself and to participate in the group play.

Daniel: In the group setting he felt more insecure than in the individual and family settings. So he somehow regressed.

Ethan: Rex's proximity-control goals and plans with respect to the others, including Gad, were easy to fathom. He wanted to get each of the children's proximity and control all of them. He tried to achieve it through the thing he was good at – soccer. If someone didn't co-operate with him, he would touch him or her in a teasing way, unless the other one ignored him completely, like Zoe. His bug was horse blinders. He didn't realize that Yuri was afraid of the ball he kicked with power. Yuri did want Rex's proximity, but from the imaginary power position of a witch, the queen of the world. Rex failed to consider that Zoe at that stage wasn't ready for any interaction. He didn't realize that he should not infringe Gad's rigid personal boundary and that his playful teasing would be interpreted by Gad as hostile rather than as friendly.

A preparatory move toward busting his horse blinders was calling him Ronaldo (the name of the soccer superstar) and styling yourself as the coach, a position of authority even over Ronaldo. You made Rex understand that he should not have approached Gad by teasing. You used illusion of alternatives by asking him whether his intention was to invite Gad to the soccer team as a goal keeper (a defensive rather than an offensive role) or as a fan. This was a way of busting Gad's non-sense, by telling him that Rex's intention was benevolent. In our previous sessions we learned that Gad used to misinterpret his peers approaches as hostile. At the same time you boosted Gad's self-image, by describing him as a brilliant future soccer player. Possible worlds. You also said that you were not sure that Gad wanted to devote himself to soccer, alluding, if I am not wrong, to his mother's attempts to mold him in her own form. You also left the door open for Gad to join Rex and the other players as a driver, a job that suits him. Gad, in his non-verbal way, looked at you, hesitating. He did not rule out the possibility of joining the play as a driver. Later he did join the play as an ambulance driver.

Shlomo: Good!

Daniel: Then Rex said the coach was ill and could not train Gad. He introduced into the play his emotive, related to his father's illness. He used transference by turning you into an image of his ill father. At the same time he dethroned you from your authority position and resumed his own control position.

Anna: You went along with that, playing the ill coach. I liked it. Sophia and Yuri immediately tried to help and heal.

Lailah: you helped Yuri overcome his fear by telling him that his magic healing power works only if he comes close, invisibly, so he's less in danger of being attacked by Rex. You reinforced his compliance by declaring that you felt better.

Ethan: Rex went back to the core of his emotive by declaring you fatally, incurably ill.

Shlomo: I said "I feel much worse, like." I added 'like' to emphasize that that was just make-believe. I thought Yuri could think I was really ill and feel scared because his magic didn't work.

Anna: Then Gad joined the play as an ambulance driver. You gathered the whole group together around you when you said that everybody should stay with you inside the ambulance, in case you would need help. You helped the group members unite around a positive goal.

Daniel: Zoe also joined in hesitantly, but still kept herself "out of the ambulance" by assuming the role of a person calling the hospital.

Shlomo: This discussion helped even me better understand my own therapeutic moves. You can see that even though the group was unstructured, each engaging in his or her own free play, a play therapist can activate play moves that achieve emotion-balancing, bug-busting and learning, tailored to the need of each member of the group.

Summary of chapter 15

Play therapy that is informed by the Diamond Model can be conducted in individual, family or group settings, simultaneously or in sequence, according to the strategy. Basically, a session, whether individual, family or group, is unstructured, although it can begin with a short, structured activity and a closing up structured activity. The participants play freely, spontaneously. The therapist observes the play and joins in as an equal play partner at a suitable moment. The therapist can be directive and initiate therapeutically relevant play moves, if spontaneous play does not happen or does not lead anywhere. The therapist does not just barge into the clients' play and imposes his or her own ideas, but attempts to fit his moves into the clients' play in a smooth, natural way. There are three kinds of play moves the therapist can make in individual, family or group play therapy. *Main moves* are designed to effect change – restoring emotion-balance related to the clients' emotives, removing or weakening bugs in the clients' intrapersonal or interpersonal programs and promoting development in relevant lines and dimensions. The role of *preparatory moves* is to prepare the ground for the main moves, getting accepted to the clients' play as an equal play partner and influencing the course of the play in ways that facilitate the activation of the main moves. *Auxiliary moves* are designed to control play acts that stand in the way of implementing a main move. There is a stock of types of preparatory moves that can be activated, but the therapist can make up his or her own preparatory moves. The types of preparatory moves have been learned by observing childrens' natural play as well as by adapting strategic techniques developed by Milton Erickson and his followers. The latter include mimicking the clients' play, pacing, focusing, the double, providing stimuli, illusion of alternatives, obedient actor and willy-nilly.

Assignments

1. Give your own examples for each of the preparatory moves: mimicking, pacing, focusing, the double, providing stimuli, illusion of alternatives, obedient actor and willy-nilly.
2. Suggest preparatory moves, auxiliary moves and main moves for individual, family and group play therapy with Case 13.2 (Bassel).

A classified list of publications

Individual play therapy

Ray, D.C. (2011). *Advanced play therapy: Essential conditions, knowledge and skills for child practice*. New York, NY: Taylor and Francis Group, LLC.

Schaefer, Ch.E. and Cangelosi, D. (2016). *Essential play therapy techniques: Time tested approaches*. New York, NY: Guilford.

Family play therapy

Ariel, S. (1994). *Strategic family play therapy*. Chichester, UK: Wiley.

Ariel, S. (1997). Strategic family play therapy. In: O'Connor, K. and Mages, L.L. eds., *Play therapy, theory and practice: A comparative casebook*. Hoboken, NJ: Wiley., pp.368–395.

Ariel, S. (2005). Family play therapy. In: Schaefer, C.J. McCormick and Ohnogi, A., eds. *The international handbook of play therapy*. New York, NY: Jason Aronson, pp.3–23.

Ariel, S., Carel, C. and Tyano, S. (1985). Uses of children's make-believe play in family therapy: Theory and clinical examples. *Journal of Marital and Family Therapy*, 11 (1), pp.47–60.

Gil, E. (1994). *Play in family therapy*. New York, NY: Guilford.

Schaefer, Ch. and Carey, L. (1994). *Family play therapy*. Northdale, NJ: Jason Aronson.

Group play therapy

Leben, N. (1993). *Directive group play therapy*. Pflugerville, TX: Morning Glory Treatment Center for Children.

O'Connor, K.J. (2001). *Group play therapy primer*. Somerset, NJ: Wiley.

Reddy, L.A. (2012). *Group play interventions for children: Strategies for teaching prosocial skills*. Washington, DC: American Psychological Association.

Sweeny, D. and Homeyer, L.E. (1999). *The handbook of group play therapy: How to do it, how it works, whom it's best for*. San Francisco, CA: Jossey-Bass.

Strategic play techniques

Erickson, M. and Rossi, E.L. (1980). *Hypnotherapy*. New York, NY: Irvington.

Madanes, C. (1991). Strategic family therapy. In: Gurman, A.S. and Kniskern D.P., eds. *Handbook of family therapy*, vol. 2. New York, NY: Guilford, pp.396–416.

Chapter 16

Lucy
The girl who created her own father

Interdisciplinary seminar

Shlomo: Today Ethan will present the case of Lucy, who he has been treating under my supervision. We'll discuss this case together.
Ethan, your turn.

Case 16.1 Lucy
Ethan: Lucy was six when her 36-year-old mother, Maya, brought her to therapy, during the summer vacation before first grade. Maya was a single mother and Lucy was her only child. Lucy was conceived by a one-night stand when Maya was on vacation in Thailand. She met Lucy's biological father in a bar. She was drunk. The man left before she woke up in her hotel room. She didn't know his name and could barely remember what he looked like. He was not a local man. He was white, Caucasian. On the same vacation she had several more such experiences. She could not remember whether she or the men had used birth control, so she was not sure that the latter was really the biological father. She decided to keep the pregnancy. She said she was plump and plain and over 30, without a chance to find a real partner. In her hometown she was lonely, with no relatives and very few female friends. She worked as a kindergarten assistant, not exactly a place where you could find single men.

When Lucy reached the age of two, she began to ask again and again, "Where is Daddy? Where is Daddy?" Maya did not know what to say to her. She told her, "far away, but he will come back". She felt very bad that she was instilling an illusion in the child's mind, but she did not think she could tell the girl the truth. Lucy wouldn't understand, and the truth would be something she could not swallow.

In the nursery school and later in the kindergarten, Lucy met children of divorced parents, but from time to time she saw a father come to take his son or daughter home. From the age of three, she completely refrained from raising the subject of the father. When Maya came to take her from kindergarten, she would tell her, "Go away!" and laugh. At home, she would slap Maya forcefully and laugh. She was crying a lot. At night she was insisting on sleeping in Maya's bed. Maya allowed her. It fulfilled her own need too. The problem was that Lucy was wetting the bed. In the kindergarten, she would start beating children without provocation and snatch away their toys.

I thought that the absence of a father explained only part of Lucy's difficulties; the loneliness of Maya and therefore of Lucy too, the interdependence between Maya and Lucy, which made it difficult for Lucy to acquire autonomy, difficulty acquiring social skills and more.

I interviewed Maya about her own history and the history of her family. I will not elaborate on this information here, because I want to concentrate on the play therapy. The pregnancy, the birth of Lucy, the milestones in her development, were normal. The intake included observing Maya and Lucy play freely together as well as observing Maya playing freely without Maya present in the room.

Here is a verbatim description of a part of the conjoint play.

Observation 16.1 Maya and Lucy

Lucy ignores me. She gives Maya a woman doll and holds a baby doll. She tells Maya, "You'll be the mommy and I'll be the baby. The baby is sleeping in the mommy's bed."

She lays the baby doll on the carpet, holds Maya's hand and almost forces her to lay the woman's doll tight against the baby doll. She says, "The baby fell asleep."

She is breathing slowly, indicating sleep.

She says, "Then the mommy turned on the darkness and did the magic that she would disappear, and the baby couldn't find her, because the mommy was already in the sky."

Maya, shocked, says, "Not true. The mommy was sleeping in the bed all night and when the baby woke, she saw her."

Maya makes the woman doll shake the baby doll's shoulder, saying, "Baby, get up, get up! Can't you see that Mama is in bed next to you?"

Lucy says, "It wasn't the real mommy. It was a doll that looked like the real mommy."

Maya says, "Not true. It was the real mommy."

Lucy throws the woman's doll across the room.

Maya looks at me, shocked. I tell her, "Don't worry, this is just play."

Lucy says, "I was inside a banana that got into my tushie and then I got soft poo, and nobody changed my diaper."

Maya (bewildered): Who was inside the banana and who wore a diaper?
Ethan: Don't look for logic. It's play.
Maya: I changed your diaper.

Lucy: You couldn't. You were far away. I made myself cornflakes with milk.
   Lucy takes a big toy bowl, tears paper into small pieces and fills two bowls with them.
Lucy: The cornflakes were for me and for the mommy.
   Lucy gets two toy spoons.
Maya (relieved): Yes, I was so hungry. Thank you for thinking about me too.
   Lucy picks up the woman doll that she had thrown, and places it next to the bowl.
   Lucy pours the contents of the bowl over the woman's doll head and laughs.
Maya: Why did you pour the cornflakes on the mommy's head?
Lucy: So, she'll eat it.
Maya: She can't eat it this way.
   Lucy picks up the woman's doll and drops it inside the bowl. She is laughing, saying, "The mommy fell into the bowl!"
Maya (smiling): The mommy likes being inside the bowl. It's nice and warm there.
   Lucy is taking the woman doll out of the bowl and pretends to eat her. She says, "Yummy!"

Anna: It's interesting that she did not introduce the father figure at all into your play and completely ignored your presence.
Daniel: This is in keeping with the fact that she had systematically stopped mentioning the father since she was three.
Ethan: She understood, at least subconsciously, that her father would never come back. She coped with this realization by ignoring his existence. She intuitively understood that if she mentioned him to Maya this would upset Maya. But wait till I describe the individual session, in which the father starred as the main protagonist.
Lailah: I saw the emotion-balancing mechanism of play in Lucy's play. Lucy's main emotive seems to be fear of being rejected and abandoned by her mother and anger at the abandoning, neglecting parent. Maybe she displaced this emotive from the father who had abandoned her to her mother. Her proximity goal was to keep the mother very close to her physically and demand of her mother to take care of her like a baby, feed her, change her diaper, etc.
   At the beginning of the play she realified contents belonging to the core of her emotive. The mother deliberately disappears when the baby is asleep. The mother was "in the sky". Dead? Then Lucy moved to contents that were less central in the associative field of the emotive. The mother couldn't change the baby's diaper because she was far away, not in the sky anymore. Later she invited the mother figure to share her corn-flakes with her, a kind of reunion.
Ethan: Throwing the mother into the bowl and then eating her was, I think, another emotion-balancing step. Swallowing the mother so that she cannot abandon.

Daniel: It shows perhaps that the very close presence of the mother was more important to Lucy than being taken care of. She can prepare food for both herself and her mother.

Lailah: Eating her was also punishing her, I think.

Ethan: It can be both keeping her close and punishing her.

Anna: I found the banana in the tushie thing bizarre and funny. I don't know what it means.

Daniel: We can say anal pleasure. We can say wishing to be back in the womb, the counterpart of swallowing . But I think these are sheer speculations.

Shlomo: I agree, but I wouldn't rule out these speculations.

Lailah: Maya's proximity-control goals were to keep Lucy close and protect her. She was very concerned about Lucy's abandonment and blaming contents. She tried to prove that she was not such a bad mother. Perhaps she felt guilty about the absence of a father. Later she accepted your explanation that this was just play. When Lucy threw the mother figure into the bowl she was amused and cooperated with the playfulness of it.

Ethan: OK, let me present a part of the individual session, which still was a part of the intake.

Session 16.1 Lucy

As soon as Lucy comes into the room, she says, "You'll be the daddy and I'll be the baby."

She is taking the baby doll she played with in the session with Maya. She is inserting it inside her T-shirt, saying, "I was the mother and the baby is in my belly. O, it hurts a little."

She takes the baby doll out of her T-shirt, saying, "Now she is being born. What a beautiful baby-princess! She's happy to be alive in the world. The daddy was the prince and he came to visit his baby princess, but on the way a ghost made him sick."

I take a man's doll to represent the father. Shlomo, according to your advice, I didn't play the father figure directly, so that the transference and Lucy's need to develop a dependent attachment to me would not be too powerful.

Lucy tells me, "Come, do as if he is sick."

I'm laying the daddy doll on the carpet, sighing, "Oh, I feel really bad."

Lucy, "And then he was dead, the daddy, and the ghost took him to the sky, because he was bad. Let's do as if you were the ghost, OK."

Ethan: Why was he bad?

Lucy: Because he always had his panties on his head.

Ethan: Why would he do that?

Lucy: Because he was bad.

Then Lucy makes the baby doll walk, as if looking for something. She is saying, "Where are my toys? All gone! The bad toy took away all the baby's toys! It even stole my beloved doll from her secret box!"

She is turning toward me and is saying, "Let's do as if the daddy punished the bad toy and gave the baby back all her toys."

I am getting a collection of toys and hand them over to the baby doll.

She is telling me, "Do you know that I am brave? Because my poop refused to get out, so I pushed and pushed, and it came out, because I am brave."

Ethan: You are really brave.

She is lying on the carpet, holding the baby doll close to her chest. She is saying, "The mommy-princess lets our baby sleep with her in the bed tonight, because she wants the baby to sleep well. The ghost came and wanted to make the mommy-princess and the daddy-prince disappear, but the baby princess crushed him like a cockroach."

Anna: Fascinating!

Daniel: When Maya wasn't in the room, she allowed herself to get her father image into the room.

Ethan: Her proximity goal was to get both her mother and her father very close to her, but both in the play with Maya and in the individual play session she fluctuated between blaming the parents for preventing her from achieving this goal and attributing this failure to external forces like "a ghost". The father wanted to visit her, but he got ill and died, because he was "bad", but then he punished the bad toy and retrieved the stolen toys. I don't know if this reflects the flip-flop bug, or the emotional-balancing mechanism of fluctuations, ups and downs.

Shlomo: It could be both.

Anna: It was funny when she said he was bad because he put his panties on his head. I think she used humor to avoid opening up the issue of anger at him because he had abandoned her.

Lailah: She was preoccupied with anal contents. The banana in the tushie, the constipation and perhaps also the panties.

Daniel: In the individual session too, her main emotive was expressed. Fear and anger at being rejected and abandoned by parental figures.

Ethan: Abandoned or being prevented by evil, punishing agents from being with her and nurturing her, getting sick, dying, disappearing, the ghost, the bad toy.

Anna: Her defenses, or emotion-balancing techniques, were regressing to babyhood and clinging to her mother, sleeping in her bed, swallowing the mother.

Daniel: Or, the contrary, she was the mother, she gave birth to the baby, she fed the mother, she got rid of the ghost by crushing it.

Lailah: From a developmental viewpoint, I think she had a problem with attachment. She could not complete the separation-individuation stage, the dimension of differentiation.

Ethan: Thank you. This discussion sharpened and clarified all kinds of thoughts I had. I won't go into the full range of information I got about this case, but will try to summarize the initial diagnostic assessment, the emotives and the related emotional imbalances, the bugs that caused Lucy inability to mobilize corrective feedback, and perhaps the developmental issue that you just referred to, Lailah. Then I'll talk about the strategy.

Initial diagnostic assessment

Emotives:

Lucy – Sadness and anger about being abandoned by her father; fear that she would be abandoned by her mother too. Also fear that her father is dead, and her mother would die too. Jealousy of children who have visible fathers.

Maya – Guilt for having raised Lucy without a father, worry and sadness with respect to the realization that Lucy doesn't trust her, doesn't acknowledge her availability and devotion.

Proximity-control goals, plans and bugs:

Lucy with respect to her father – seeking his proximity and protection, imagining him coming and protecting her, or prevented from coming by external agents and unable to protect her.

Main bug – horse blinders. She had no information about her father or the possibility of his arrival someday.

This bug prevents her from getting corrective feedback and is related to the question of whether she should hope for him to be a part of her life in the future or if she should abandon hope and go through a real process of mourning.

Lucy with respect to Maya – seeking her physical proximity, by clinging and controlling her so she won't leave.

Bugs –

fifth wheel. The absence of her mother is irrelevant to the presence or absence of her father.

Horse blinders. She withheld information from her mother about her thoughts and feelings concerning the absence of her father. She didn't re-examine her supposition that her mother would be upset if she mentioned her father.

Maybe flip-flop, as she fluctuated between controlling and controlled positions with respect to her mother.

These bugs prevented her from mobilizing corrective feedback, gaining clear information about her father and obtaining reassurance that her mother would not abandon her.

Maya with respect to Lucy – keeping her close. Maybe over-protecting her. Reassuring her that she is available and won't abandon her.

Bugs –
horse blinders. She co-operated with Lucy's silence about her father. She didn't see the connection between that and Lucy' anxiety concerning her motherhood. This bug prevented her from getting corrective feedback about Lucy's state of mind and about what can be done to reassure her.

Developmentally, maybe Lucy had an arrested separation-individuation process.

Strategy

Shlomo: Ethan and I discussed the question of whether it would advisable and desirable that Maya told Lucy the truth about her father. Both of us had a feeling, somewhat ambiguous and not fully decisive, that Lucy was not ripe and ready to know the truth and come to terms with it. The question was whether the truth really would allow her to start a healthy process of mourning, or rather put her in a state of distress that would increase her emotive-related emotional imbalance, fortify her bugs and cause her to regress more deeply into inability to continue the separation-individuation process.

Anna: I wouldn't tell her the truth at this stage.

Lailah: I would. Lucy strikes me as a very intelligent and sensitive girls. Deep inside, as we already said, she knew the truth. Confirming her intuitive knowledge, however difficult and bitter, would help her cope better and mobilize resilience, I think.

Daniel: I feel ambivalent. I have no clear opinion.

Ethan: Anyway, we decided not to break this news to her yet. A part of the strategy we decided on was co-operating with Lucy in building a presence of a father figure in the imaginative make-believe play world and helping Maya to take part in this process, which would all happen within the play world. The owning and alienation would prevent Lucy from cultivating false hopes. It would help her derive emotional satisfaction from an imaginary relationship with the father figure without deluding herself that this is a current or future reality.

In accordance with the strategy we decided upon, at the beginning of the therapy Lucy would participate in individual play sessions, designed to help her reach an emotive-related emotional balance and weaken or remove the horse blinders bugs in her proximity plan with respect to her imagined father. The individual sessions should come first, because the presence of her mother would probably block and inhibit her working through the father issue. In the second stage, Lucy and Maya would participate together in dyadic play sessions, whose purposes would be to help both of them re-balance their emotive-related emotions and weaken the bugs in their proximity-control plans. The father figure and everything related to it would be fully present at these sessions. Maya and Lucy would create a present, protective and functioning father, albeit only in the pretend world of the play.

Anna: Isn't that a bit risky? Is there no danger that Lucy, despite the owning and alienation, would over-indulge in this fantasy on the one hand and on the other hand find it even more difficult to come to terms with the bitter reality?

Shlomo: There is such danger indeed, but Lucy did give the father figure a prominent place in her make-believe play anyway. Every therapy should be conducted with caution. If the play would seem to take Lucy to undesirable places, we could always change direction.

Ethan: I'll now present two vignettes. One from an individual session with Lucy and the other one from a session with both Lucy and Maya.

Session 16.2 Lucy

Lucy holds a wooden stick and paints it in pastel colors. She is saying, without looking at me, "I am preparing a magic wand. You will be the evil sorcerer and I will be the good magician. You will plan to make the palace disappear and I will use my magic so that it will not disappear."

I am putting on a black sorcerer's conical hat and am chanting, "Palace, disappear! Palace, disappear!"

Lucy is stretching out her arm with the magic wand toward me, shakes the magic wand and says, "Palace, don't disappear! Palace, don't disappear! It didn't disappear, but it is invisible, and the sorcerer cannot see it."

I laugh wickedly and say, "It's gone, it disappeared."

I am addressing Lucy, "The evil sorcerer didn't know that the palace didn't vanish, because the magician made it transparent and he couldn't see it."

Lucy picks up the baby doll she played with in the previous sessions. She says, "The baby can see the palace, but his mother-princess will not allow him to get in because he is stinking of poo."

I say, "Let's pretend the mother-princess can smell everything but she cannot smell the baby's poo, so she lets him in".

Lucy: She didn't change his diaper because she didn't smell his poo and she didn't know he was dirty.

Ethan: I am taking the man's doll from the previous sessions. I say, "The daddy changed the baby's diaper".

Lucy: He didn't, because the smell made him sick and he ran away.

Ethan: I make the man's doll run away, saying, "The smell of the baby's poo made me sick."

Lucy is taking a dog's toy. She says, "The stink made the dog sick too because he has a very strong sense of smell".

I say, "Let's play as if the dog ate the daddy's nose and this made the dog sick."

Lucy likes the idea. She makes the dog bite the man's nose.

I say, "Now the daddy-prince had no sense of smell because the dog ate his nose, so he couldn't smell the poo, so he came back to the palace and helped the mother-princess change the baby's diaper, because he saw the poo even though he couldn't smell it. And then both the daddy and the mommy cleaned the baby's tushie with a tissue and spread an ointment on it."

Lucy "buys" this idea. We play as if the man's doll and Lucy change the baby doll diaper, clean it and spread ointment on it.

Lucy: And then the sorcerer made the daddy and the mommy disappear.
Ethan: But the magician cancelled the spell with his magic wand.

Lucy is throwing the "magic wand" away. She is lying on her back and is crying like a baby. I make the man's doll come close to her and touch her shoulder, saying "Why are you crying, my baby princess. Daddy is here."

She continues crying for a while. Then she is getting up, taking a clown doll and makes it dance and sing, "I am the funny clown! I don't scare the kids! I just make them laugh!"

She puts the clown under a table, makes him continue dancing and repeating these verses. She says, "The clown is dancing inside the fridge, but he is not cold, because he is dancing."

Lailah: Like with the panties on the father's head, one of her emotion-balancing technique is resorting to funny, "silly" contents to calm herself down.
Daniel: We see in this session other manifestations of her main emotive, fear of being abandoned by parental figures. The palace that disappears, the father and mother who disappeared, the father who ran away.
Anna: When you borrowed her idea of the magician undoing with his magic wand the spell that made the father and mother disappear, she threw the magic wand away and cried like a baby, as if saying, "I don't believe that the father and mother will stay or be retrieved," and then she expressed her helplessness and distress as an abandoned baby.
Lailah: As in the previous sessions, she attributed the disappearance or departure of the father and mother figures either to evil external forces, in this case the sorcerer, or to the parental figures' free will – the father who ran away because he couldn't stand the smell of the baby's poo and it made him sick.
Daniel: There is a new element here, blaming herself for the father's escape, her bad smell. We see again the anal content popping up over and over again in her play.
Anna: We see again the various emotion-balancing techniques she was using: the magic wand, the palace becoming invisible so that the sorcerer cannot see it, and also moving from contents close to the core of her emotive to funny, "silly" contents like the clown dancing inside the fridge.
Daniel: The emotion-balancing technique of fluctuations (ups and downs) is manifested in this vignette too. She goes from the core of her emotive to its periphery, then outside of the emotive's associations field and back to the core.
Ethan: How would you interpret my play-therapeutic interventions?
Anna: First you went with her realified contents, not against them, and elaborated them. I like it. You made your own emotion-balancing moves, like saying,

"She can smell everything, but she cannot smell the baby's poo, so she lets him in."

Ethan: I assumed that her proximity plan with respect to her mother and imaginary father were infected with horse blinders and non-sense. She suspected that they didn't want her because she was disgusting or something like that. In this intervention I used the bug busters owning and alienation and basic duality, implying that even if she owns her being disgusting, it is only make-believe, and she can be alienated from it. And I also implied that a mother, any mother, including her own mother, cannot be really disgusted by her baby's feces, because she is her baby and she loves her.

Daniel: When she said, "She didn't smell his poo and she didn't know he was dirty." You said, "The daddy changed his diaper." You turned the imagined father into a nurturing, responsible parent.

Ethan: Yes, in this and my later interventions I used the bug-buster possible worlds, to help Lucy create an imaginary fully functioning and present father, in accordance with the strategy we decided on. At first she didn't go along with this idea, made the daddy feel sick and run away. I used pacing. I did run away, but then gradually came back. Then she collaborated with me in changing the diaper, even though it was just for a short while. This was a possible world in which both the mother and the father co-operated in nurturing the baby. For her this was emotionally satisfying.

Anna: Lucy likes funny, absurd ideas, and you associated with her in this respect by saying that the dog ate the daddy's nose and got sick, but the daddy wasn't sick anymore and came back to change the baby's diaper.

Daniel: Perhaps at the same time it also satisfied Lucy's need to punish her father for abandoning her.

Ethan: It's really good that we're having this conversation. It is encouraging. I begin to understand my intuitive moves in doing the play therapy.

I am going to now present a vignette from a dyadic session with Lucy and Maya. Before that, there had been a few more individual meetings with Lucy, in which she talked about "ghosts who kidnapped the daddy". I invented a body called "Daddies Finders", a kind of agency whose function was to search for missing daddies, and if necessary, to rescue them. I was the director of that agency. I used a large anatomical doll, employed in child abuse investigations, that could serve as a kind of identi-kit. It was a large cloth doll, without any hair, facial parts or gender identity body parts. One could attach to its face eyes, eye-lashes, a nose, ears, eyebrows lips, head and facial hair or stubble, from a given large selection. It was also possible to dress it in clothes, put on it shoes and a hat, all from a large selection.

I told her that in order to find the father we needed to know what he looked like, to identify him. She made a figure of a man with fair curly hair, blue eyes with long eyelashes, bushy eyebrows, fleshy nose, thick smiling lips and prominent ears. He looked a little bit like a clown, reminded me of Harpo Marx. She dressed him in jeans and a T-shirt and made him wear white shoes. She also put a red plastic heart in a little box and wrapped the box with a paper. She placed the box under his arm and said that it was a gift he would give the girl when he came back home. Then we played scenes of looking for the daddy, finding him, rescuing him, homecoming and joining the family. In all these scenes the daddy played with the girl (she wasn't a baby anymore), but then he was kidnapped by the ghosts again and the cycle, finding, rescuing, homecoming, etc. was repeated. She insisted on playing this scene over and over again, in all the sessions.

I prepared Maya for the dyadic sessions. I told her about the daddy figure and the repeated homecoming scene. We decided that she would take an active part in this play. Let me present the dyadic session and then we'll discuss it.

Session 16.3 Maya and Lucy
Lucy is already in first grade. She is drawing a big blue heart on the whiteboard and writes "Daddy", "Mommy", "Lucy" inside it and then immediately rubs the picture out.

I get the daddy doll from the previous individual sessions and make it stand in front of Maya and Lucy. Maya is saying, "Oh, here is the daddy!" Lucy says, "It's only a doll". She angrily strips the doll of everything, throwing each item on the carpet, until what remains is the naked doll without any clothes or human features. Maya looks upset and doesn't know how to respond.

I say, "Lets make-believe the daddy was a doll".

Lucy doesn't respond.

Maya says, "Can I turn the doll into a person?" Lucy does not respond. Maya says, "I will not turn the doll into daddy, I'll turn it into a person".

Lucy is going to the box of costumes. She chooses a clown's costume, including hair, and starts disguising herself.

Maya begins dressing the doll and attaching to it facial parts and features – straight black hair, brown eyes and eyebrows, prominent nose, wide lips, stubble and a suit, attempting to create a manly, attractive man.

Lucy, disguised as a clown, stands in front of her and starts dancing violently, making grimaces and loud noises.

I say, "I am the circus manager. The man and the woman came to see the show. Let's pretend that the clown tried to entertain and amuse them."

Lucy stop dancing and shouting. She comes closer to Maya and says, "He does not look like the Daddy at all."

Maya says, "He is another daddy. He took us to the circus."

Lucy says, "The daddy was an acrobat. He walked on a rope and fell and got a painful blow."

I take a man's doll and makes it fall on the carpet. I cry, "Emergency! Our acrobat fell and got a painful blow! Clown, Mommy, Man, come and help him!"

Maya and Lucy, as the clown, bend over the "acrobat" and help him get up.

I say, "Our clown is a doctor. He is both a doctor and a clown."

Lucy says, "The doctor says that he will be alright."
Maya says, "Let's take him home. Do we need an ambulance?"
I say, "No, he can walk."
I say, as the daddy-acrobat, "Daddy is OK. Daddy can even teach you how to stand on your head."
Lucy is saying, "I know how to stand on my head!"
She is trying to demonstrate this but falls.
I am saying as the daddy doll, "Try again, Mommy will hold your legs. One day you will be an acrobat like Daddy."

Anna: In contrast to the individual meetings, when Lucy was with her mother, most of the time she resisted admitting the father's figure into the play. She immediately erased the drawing of the heart with the father, the mother and herself inside. She said that the father figure she created was only a doll and tore out angrily all his identifying features. She rejected the man's doll Maya created and tried to hinder Maya from creating that character by playing the role of the wild clown. Like in previous sessions, she caused the father figure (the "acrobat") to fall and get hurt. She could accept him only when he was weak and vulnerable. Only toward the end of the session could she accept him as her trainer.

Ethan: I think that was because the mother's presence still aroused in her mistrust and anger. She still, deep inside, blamed Maya, and also indirectly the father, for her having been abandoned. Perhaps she was angry at me too, for forcing her not to continue avoiding the father's issue in her mother's presence.

Lailah: Maya created the man she would like to have as a partner. Handsome, manly. This make-believe play was emotionally satisfying for her too.

Daniel: I liked it that you encouraged Lucy to create her own concrete father figure. She created a soft figure, not threatening. And in the session with Maya you encouraged her to continue developing this character. You didn't say anything, just showed the doll she made.

Anna: When Lucy stripped her father figure and said it was just a doll, you said, "Let's make-believe the daddy was a doll!" Why did you say it?

Ethan: First of all, I didn't contradict her. But by saying it I activated two bug-busters – owning and alienation and arbitrariness of the signifier. Thanks to the denial of seriousness, what I said implied, "The daddy was not a doll." She could both own and disown the idea that the doll represented a father figure. Also, I implied that the doll was an arbitrary signifier for the father figure, even though he was stripped of visible human features.

Shlomo: An excellent application of the concepts you have learned.

Daniel: When Lucy played the clown, you said, "I am the circus manager, the man and the woman came to see the show. Let's pretend that the clown tried to entertain and amuse them." First you used the willy-nilly technique by assuming the authoritative role of the circus manager, which suited Lucy's clown role. You reframed Lucy's control plan of interfering with Maya's attempt to create her own male figure, by re-defining this control plan as a benevolent effort to accept Maya and her own male figure and entertain them. You called them "the man and the woman", not "the daddy and the mommy", respecting Lucy's refusal to accept the male figure as a daddy. It was Maya that said "He is another daddy", and it was Lucy who agreed to see him as the father, and said, "The daddy is an acrobat. He walked on the rope and fell and got a painful blow."

Lailah: Then you turned the injured daddy-acrobat into a strong parental figure, who can teach Lucy his trade. She went along with this idea. I see that Lucy was ready to accept a father figure into her play it he met her real needs, even if she had previously rejected that father figure.

Shlomo:I would like to commend Ethan for his excellent therapeutic work. You succeeded in combining creativity, systematic thinking and understanding of the concepts of The Diamond Model. I would like to commend all of you for having internalized The Diamond Model and for your ability to speak in the theoretical language you have learned.

Summary of chapter 16

This chapter is devoted to illustrating the model detailed in this book, by presenting a case of a single mother, Maya, and her six-year-old daughter Lucy. The mother was not sure who the father was and there was no way to find him. Lucy stopped asking Maya "Where is daddy?" since she was three. She intuitively understood that the father would not come and did not want to upset her mother by raising the issue. She developed symptoms such as clinging to her mother, bed-wetting and aggression directed at Maya and at peers. The question asked by Maya as well as by the members of the interdisciplinary seminar was whether Lucy should have been told the truth or not. Pros and cons were discussed. The therapist, Ethan, consulted me as his supervisor. We both decided that it was too early to break the news to Lucy. The strategy chosen was to help Lucy create her own make-believe father figure and realify it in her make-believe world, first in individual play therapy sessions and later in dyadic sessions with Maya. Vignettes from the individual and dyadic play therapy sessions were discussed in the interdisciplinary seminar.

Assignments

1. Discuss the pros and cons of telling Lucy the truth about her father vs. letting her create her own make-believe father figure.
2. Suggest an alternative strategy for Case 16.1 (Lucy) and five alternative play-therapeutic moves in an individual session with Lucy and in a dyadic session with Lucy and Maya.

A classifies list of publications

Play therapy with children of a single-parent family

Ariel, S. (1992). *Strategic family play therapy*. Chichester, UK: Wiley.
Bratton, S. and Landreth, G. (1995). Filial therapy with single parents: Effects on parental acceptance, empathy, and stress. *International Journal of Play Therapy*, 4 (1), pp.61–80.

Chapter 17

Nadav
A sweet oppositional-defiant boy

Case 17.1 Nadav

The parents of ten-year-old Nadav, their only child, sit in my office. His father Menashe, an unkempt, unshaven 45-year-old man, looks at me with a permanently angry facial expression. His mother Amalia, a big, overweight 38-year-old woman, is looking at him, waiting for him to speak. He doesn't say anything, so she turns to me and says, "Nadav is a good boy, charming. He tells himself lots of things inside and takes it all out on me."

*Me*nashe: Every exchange between Amalia and Nadav ends up in a fight. A Fourth World War. "Nadav, stop playing with your stupid computer games and do your homework!"; "Nadav, take a shower and brush your teeth!"; "Nadav, clean all the mess you've made all over the apartment!" His response is, "Shut up! If you go on talking, I'll give you trouble! I'll turn your life into hell!"

The same thing in school, he is disobedient and impudent with the teachers, does just what he wants, learns only when he feels like it. His notebooks and writing tools are in a mess.

Until recently I had been restraining him, but now I got tired and gave up. I've taken three steps backwards. If I punish him, there will not be anyone to put the pieces together.

Amalia: He blames me for things he is the one who is responsible for. He did something wrong with his computer? "Why did you damage my computer?" He forgot to recharge his smartphone? "Why did you pull out the chord?"

I used to take him places to have a good time with me, but what he wanted was always only that I buy him things, and if I refused, he was very angry and wanted to go home, so I stopped taking him places.

Menashe: He always tries to extort us, computer games, electric bicycle and so on, and would never give anything in return. I tear myself apart to bring bread home and he does not appreciate it. Thinks he deserves everything. He is the king, and we are his slaves.

Amalia: The kids like him, but he cannot tolerate not being on top. He was in a soccer club, but when he saw that he wasn't accepted as the leader, number one, he left the club, said he didn't like it.

Later in the interview, the parents told me that Nadav's development was normal, but a few months before the start of therapy he was diagnosed with ADHD and with significant gaps in cognitive and psychomotor abilities. His behavior problems started when he was in first grade.

Amalia grew up in a normative family. She also was diagnosed with ADHD. As a child she had many medical problems. She didn't want to go to school and barely finished elementary school. Presently she is healthy and works as a cashier in a supermarket.

Menashe grew up with a volatile Holocaust survivor father, who was aggressive and often violent. He described life in his childhood home as hell. He refused to go to school, would spend most of his time on the streets. His father left home when he was nine. Menashe was placed in a therapeutic boarding facility, but he left it and lived in a tent in a forest. His father moved to a Kibbutz.

When Amalia was pregnant, the family moved to live with a sister of Amalia's grandmother, who was a solitary Holocaust survivor. She was like a mother to Nadav and had been like a mother to Amalia. She used to play and have a good time with Nadav. Her health began deteriorating when Nadav was five. She died when he was six. Outwardly, the loss didn't seem to have an impact on Nadav, but Amalia said she knew that deep inside he took it very hard. At the same year Menashe suffered from serious medical problems and spent almost the whole year in hospitals. Amalia was depressed, had to work extra time. Nadav was left to his own devices.

The therapy started toward the end of Nadav's summer vacation, between his fifth and sixth grades.

Interdisciplinary seminar

Ethan: Menashe has an angry look and seems to be an aggressive disciplinarian.
Daniel: And the fact that he gave up trying to discipline Nadav.
Lailah: I am asking myself whether Nadav's oppositional-defiant behavior and his low functioning weren't caused mainly by his ADHA and his uneven cognitive-emotional profile. His behavior difficulties began when he started first grade.
Shlomo: Let me remind you, Lailah, that the Diamond Model is multi-systemic. There is never just one cause to the difficulties we are called for to treat.
Ethan: We shouldn't forget that before the time Nadav started first grade, his old mother-substitute died and his father was absent because of medical problems.
Shlomo: You are right.

OK, let me present the first play session with Nadav and his parents.

Observation 17.1 Nadav, Menashe and Amalia
Nadav looks different from what I expected. Plump, cuddly, jumpy, sparks in his eyes and a big smile.

At the beginning of the session, the family participated in a play activity that I often conduct in such sessions. Each family member chooses a puppet from a given collection, gives it a name, makes up and enacts a story that includes the other puppets.

Amalia chose a big teddy-bear puppet and called it Poopy. She said that Poopy was her nickname for Menashe. The latter chose a dinosaur puppet and called it Zaur. Nadav was very enthusiastic. He was laughing excitedly. He chose a cow puppet and called it Moo-Moo. He pounced upon Poopy and began chewing and hitting it.

Amalia, laughing said, "Hi Moo-Moo! Why are you eating up Poopy?"

Nadav, moving fast, turned toward Zaur and made Moo-Moo hit and bite Zaur. He said, "Moo-Moo is killing and eating everybody".

I said, "OK, Amalia's story".

Amalia: Once there were three friends, Zaur, Poopy and Moo-Moo. They were spending all day together. And then Moo-Moo got crazy and started fighting with Poopy.

Nadav made Moo-Moo hit and bite Zaur and said, "Zaur is dead!"

Menashe's story: Three million years ago, all the dinosaurs were extinct. Only one was left, Zaur. He began looking for friends. He came across an annoying cow, Moo-Moo, who didn't want to be his friend. Then Moo-Moo killed Zaur and was left alone, lonely.

Nadav hit Zaur with Moo-Moo, shouting, "Big mouth! I'm going to eat you up!" Then he said, "Moo-Moo fought Zaur and Poopy in five championships and won in all of them, and then she killed all the contestants. She wanted to have friends, but she was too hungry all the time, so she ate them all up. She got a stomach ache, but she preferred them inside her tummy, because this way they couldn't get on her nerves. Inside her tummy they just tickled.

Then Nadav lay down on the carpet, apparently exhausted.

Anna: It's nice to see how the owning and alienation of play allow the participants to express difficult contents related to their inner world and their relationships yet remain in an amused mood. The play had an ameliorating effect. It helped them achieve emotional balance.

Suddenly I felt empathy toward Menashe. He expressed his terrible loneliness, his desperate need for love and his deep disappointment that Nadav was denying him that love. He also expressed sincere empathic concern, that Nadav sabotaged the possibility of receiving love from his parents and was therefore doomed to loneliness.

Amalia also felt a need to win Nadav's love. She expressed her inability to understand why he didn't give her the kind of love she gave him. In her mind, there was no reason for that. Nadav just went crazy. That was her horse blinders, but how could she know what kinds of devils inhabited Nadav's mind?

Lailah: It's interesting that Amalia gave her puppet a name that's the same as her husband's nickname. It's like she didn't differentiate between Menashe and herself.

Anna: So, when Nadav attacked Poopy he attacked both his parents.

Daniel: She chose a bear toy. You said she was a big woman.

Shlomo: All three of them were overweight.

Lailah: Interestingly, Nadav chose a predator cow. He was aggressive, but you said that he was a smiling, cuddly boy. It is as if he wanted to give the message, "I am angry, but deep inside I am soft".

Shlomo: Yes, the choice of toys is never coincidental.

Daniel: Nadav said that Moo-Moo did want to have friends, but she ate up all her friends because she was hungry all the time. He said that inside Moo-Moo's tummy they wouldn't get on her nerves. This reminds me of fantasies of swallowing and cannibalism in some psychoanalytic theories, Melanie Klein's for instance. It is a combination of aggression and desire to keep the parental figure inside by introjection. Once he has his parents inside him, he will have them all for himself, control them and stop feeling a victim of their aggression. This is related to his omnipotence defense. He kills all the contestants. As Amalia said, he has to be on top all the time.

Shlomo: Yes. Swallowing and devouring fantasies are discussed by Melanie Klein and other psychoanalysis (see for instance Klein, 1957). And also by ethno-psychiatrists who studied myths of cannibalism in various cultures (see for instance Hiatt, 1975).

Anna: Lucy also played as if she ate up her mother (Case 16.1).

Ethan: Nadav's proximity-control programs with respect to his parents seem to be infected with horse blinders, fifth wheel and non-sense. He could see only what he wrongly interpreted as their negative attitude toward him. His bugs were energized by great anger. We have to uncover the sources of his anger. Maybe it had to do with the year he had lost the woman who treated him like a mother, the year his father was ill and his mother was depressed. That was a crisis that caused him severe emotional distress and loss of the simplicity of his previous plans. He maintained partial simplicity – consistency at the expense of comprehensiveness; failing to see the overall picture – horse blinders; consistent lack of basic trust in his parents' love at the cost of parsimony, lack of awareness of the irrelevance of the crisis five years earlier to his current life situation – fifth wheel; consistency at the cost of plausibility, misinterpreting his parents' responses. All that resulted in inability to enlist corrective feedback, an escalating amplified deviation from homeostasis. There were of course many other influencing factors, e.g. his scholastic difficulties, his ADAD and perhaps his father's angry temper and his difficult past. So, we need to help him re-balance his emotive-related emotions and bust his bugs by play bug-busters.

Shlomo: Amalia told me that when Nadav entered first grade he started misbehaving in school and refused to participate in any learning activities. She and her husband thought he was just lazy and insolent and didn't understand his difficulties. They were angry at him, yelling at him quite often. Once Menashe, in front of his peers and some shocked parents, pulled his ear, quite painfully, and shouted, "You listen to me, can you hear me?!" Amalia withheld this information from me until a later stage of the therapy, too ashamed to share it with me right from the beginning. Here is one of the sources of Nadav's anger, Ethan.

Anna: And that was after he lost his mother-substitute and almost lost his father. I feel so sorry for him!

Lailah: I'm not sure Nadav preserved consistency so rigidly. He seems to be ambivalent with respect to his parents.

Shlomo: I think the next session will largely confirm your insightful analyses.

Let's consider the first individual play therapy session with Nadav.

Session 17.1 Nadav

Amalia brought Nadav. He refused to enter the apartment that serves as my clinic. After ten minutes of entreaties and threats, Amalia was about to give in and take him back home, but at that point he agreed to enter. He brought a ball with him and began kicking it, running around the apartment. I decided not to stop him by exercising my authority. That's exactly what he expected me to do. Instead, I suggested having him do a psychological test. This aroused his curiosity. He agreed to enter, not the large room where I do family and group play therapy, but the smaller room where I do individual and couple therapy with adults and psychological tests. I showed him some pictures of the TAT projective test and asked him to tell stories inspired by these pictures.

His story for the first picture, which depicts a little boy sitting alone in the entrance of a hut:

"Once there were two brothers and a mother. The Nazis came to their home and killed their mother, and the British soldiers killed his brother. He was left alone, never married, had no job, had no money, borrowed some money from his grandfather, had no friends, had nothing in his life. That's what this picture looks like."

A picture of an old woman and a young man:

"Queen Elisabeth refused to give her son the money she inherited from her dead father. His grandfather, the king, had been the richest man in the world. Queen Elisabeth quarreled with her son about fifty trillion gold coins. She said, 'You are too young to get the money'. He was angry, and she said, 'I don't know what to do with him'."

A picture of men resting in a field:

"Four people ran away from a murderer. He almost got them, but the police caught them and he got a life sentence."

A picture of a boy looking forward. Behind him a man lying on a bed, seems to be operated on by people:

"This boy is hiding from the men in the previous picture. His brother was the murderer who wanted to kill them."

(Nadav ignored the back scene.)

A picture of a man with hands holding him from behind:

"A Hollywood star. He borrowed money from loan sharks. He didn't pay his debt. They caught him. He fought them and won, until one of them shot him in the back and he died."

A picture of a woman sitting on the floor with her back to the viewer of the picture:

"Miss Berger was a lonely woman. Already during her childhood, she had a horrible face. Nobody wanted to stay near her. Only her brother could tolerate her. When she grew up, she had no work and was always alone. She was the laughing stock of people, because of her ugly face, and then she died."

A picture of an older man and a younger man:

"Once there was the son of the Prime Minister. He had a big nose, and everybody mocked him. His father said, 'Whoever is making fun of you will die'."

A picture of a boy looking at a violin:

"He was the class nerd. He was very intelligent, but he wasn't good at math. He said, 'One plus one is one'. The children used to make fun of him. He dropped out of school and was alone and unemployed all his life."

A picture of a shadow of a boy in a window:

"There was a boy who was very angry at his mother. He wanted to commit suicide. He jumped out of the window and died."

A picture of a woman looking into a room:

"This woman makes me feel uneasy. She has the most disturbing face in the whole world. Everybody used to mock her, the whole neighborhood, the whole city, the whole universe. She locked herself inside her home until she was old and died."

(The woman in the picture has a nice face, with a worried expression.)

Anna: What a tormented soul! I feel so sorry for him. I don't know, his stories contain themes from the Second World War, as well as a lot of blood and murders. Amalia said that he had lived with a Holocaust survivor. His grandfather on his father's side was a Holocaust survivor. We know of third generation Holocaust survivors' syndromes.

Shlomo: Almost all Israeli children, Jews and Arabs, live in a war-stricken country and are exposed to stories about the Holocaust.

Let's concentrate on the question of what the main emotives expressed in his story are.

Lailah: Hopelessness, doomed to a life of misery, loneliness, poverty, being rejected by society.

Shlomo: This is the general pessimistic picture. Can you discern specific emotives?

Daniel: Mourning the loss of a brother and a mother. The brother was killed in war, or, in another story, imprisoned for life.

The only one who could tolerate the face of the woman was her brother. The brother image was the only relatively positive figure in the protagonist's life. Apparently, the protagonist is Nadav's representation of his own self.

Ethan: But the father figure, who is mentioned only once, protected him by threatening the people who were making fun of him.

Anna: Nadav, as an only child who doesn't get along with his parents, was yearning for a brother.

Lailah: Loneliness. No family, no friends.

Ethan: Shame related to physical appearance. Ugly, disturbing, deterring face, causing the person to be the laughing stock of people, and therefore doomed to a life of seclusion and loneliness.

Daniel: But only of a woman's face. Does he allude to his own face, or perhaps to his mother's face?

Lailah: Maybe he projected on her "the bad mother" internal objects.

Anna: Not only a woman's face. The king's son had a long nose and was ridiculed by people.

Daniel: Fear of being killed, murdered.

Ethan: No job, poverty. Denied his grandfather's inheritance. Bitterness.

I'm asking myself whether this is related to his parents' refusal to buy him whatever he demands. He believes he deserves everything he demands. Horse blinders.

Anna: Shame for learning difficulties. Being ridiculed not just because of his face but also because he is not good at math. Probably this is related to his ADHD and his uneven cognitive profile.

Shlomo: By the way, Nadav is very good at math.

Lailah: Upset because of his fights with his mother. Has suicidal ideation, because he sees no way out of their mutual bickering.

Daniel: The suicidal ideation was related not just to his relationship with his parents. His whole world view was extremely pessimistic.

Ethan: I wonder if we can arrange all these in a single CDCA chart.

Shlomo: Maybe, but let's not do it now. I'd like to present to you more vignettes.

Session 17.2 Nadav

After having completed the TAT test, Nadav himself suggested to go and play in the larger play therapy room. He immediately started to search the room. All the toys and play things were not openly displayed, but were inside drawers in a cabinet. He pulled out the drawers without asking for permission and took out various toys representing biting or stinging creatures such as scorpions, snakes and spiders.

He said, "I'll take these homes and hide them in my mother's bed".

I didn't respond. I was sure he knew I wouldn't let him take them home.

He said, "you stand here".

He took out toys representing various birds of prey. He gave me the biting-stinging creatures and kept the birds of prey. Then he made the birds of prey pounce on the biting-stinging creatures.

He says, "They killed them all, but before they were dead, they had stung the birds with their venom and all the birds died except for one eagle".

He made an eagle toy fly above the dead birds and said, "The eagle revived all of them with his wings".

He pointed at the biting-stinging creatures and told me, "Make them move! Make them move!" I moved them. He said, "They didn't really die, they only fainted".

He resumed the battle between birds of prey the biting-stinging creatures.

He said, "Now the birds really killed all of them. But now the birds start killing each other".

He made the birds of prey attack each other and they all fell on the carpet, dead.

He got two large toy dogs and said, "These were the Doom Doom twin brothers. Their parents were killed by the stinging creatures and the birds of prey when they were little. They had no choice. They had to learn to fight to survive".

Lailah: He played like a five or six-year-old boy. From my experience, children of his age don't usually play such make-believe scenes.

Daniel: He began to be problematic toward the age of six, when his substitute mother died, his father was ill and absent and later he was treated harshly by his parents. He went back there because he had some issues to resolve and work through.

Shlomo: An interesting hypothesis.

Ethan: Some of the themes included in his TAT stories appear in his play too. Murderous aggression. Everybody is killed except one.

Lailah: He did use, minimally, some emotion-balancing techniques, such as reversal.

Anna: But then the birds of prey, who were supposed to be loyal to each other, killed each other. Is this related to his unresolved power struggle with his parents, especially his mother? In one of his TAT stories, the boy committed suicide because he didn't get along with his mother.

Lailah: The brother theme again. The Doom Doom brothers. Their parents were murdered when they were little. It seems like this is also related to the loss of his substitute mother and the absence of his father, who was in a life danger. Then he developed a life script: Even though I am only a child, I am alone in this world and I have to fight to survive, like a lone wolf.

Ethan: As I said, preserving consistency at the cost of parsimony, comprehensiveness and plausibility. His omnipotence defense, his self-reliance, was reinforced by his parents' bugged control plans in response to his oppositional-defiant behavior and school problems. They were fluctuating between angry, aggressive responses and helplessness. Horse blinders. flip-flop. They didn't understand what we begin to understand. Their bugs should be busted by bug-busters. In order to achieve this, one should help them re-balance their emotions of frustration and anger. Of course, Nadav's behavior toward them was also bugged.

Shlomo: Here is another individual session with Nadav:

Session 17.3 Nadav

Nadav enters the apartment, fuming, and locks the entrance door behind him. He says, "Don't let my mother in, and if you let her in, I'm going to make sure she stays outside."

I ignore his warning. I open the door and let Amalia in. Nadav doesn't say anything. Amalia is waiting in the smaller room. Once in the play therapy room, Nadav explains that he is angry at Amalia because she didn't let him cross a road on his scooter.

I say, "You are angry because she doesn't rely on you to take care of your own safety, and she is too worried, as if you are a little kid."

He says, "Exactly."

He looks restless. He says that he is bored and asks me if I have computer games. I say I don't. He asks me if he can go home. I say he can. He doesn't move.

After a while he takes a wizard's hat out of a box and puts it on. I wear another wizard's hat and say, "We are both wizards." He says he can transform people into predators. I say I can turn predators into good people.

I say, "Bad wolf, bad wolf, I'm going to turn you into a good granny".

I take off the wizard's hat, put on a gray-haired woman's wig, and talk to him like a loving grandmother. I say, "My wizard, I'm your grandma. I love you so much! Do you remember how I taught you to be a wizard? I taught you all the tricks of the trade."

He says angrily, "I'm going to turn you into a bad wolf again!"

I put on the magician's hat and ask him why he threatened to transform her to a bad wolf. He says, "I didn't like the way she was talking. She should have howled like a wolf."

I make the old woman reappear and howl at him.

He says, "You are not grandma, you are a wolf disguised as grandma. You devoured grandma."

I say, "I am the chief magician in a magicians' school and you are the best teacher in my school. I'll turn the wolf into a real grandma and you'll teach her how to be a good magician, who knows exactly how to talk as a magician should talk."

He says he will turn her into a wolf again, because she devoured her two children.

I take a transparent plastic ball and look through it. I say that I can see in my crystal ball what really happened. It wasn't she who devoured the two children, but a bad wolf.

He says, "Your crystal ball is false. The woman replaced your crystal ball with a false one. She is a bad witch who pretends to be a good magician."

I say, the bad witches planted this idea in your mind. I'm going to use my magic to remove the spell. Then you will remember what really happened. I will also give you some trust potion."

He lies down on the carpet, looking exhausted. He says, "I'm five-years-old, no, ten, no, five-years-old."

I say, "Let's play as if now is then, the time when you were five."

He says, "When I was five-years-old I didn't get enough attention, so I became more and more tough."

I look through the transparent ball and say, "I see in my crystal ball two figures, a five-year-old boy and a ten-year-old boy. Then they merge and become one person."

I give him a plastic glass and tell him to drink some trust potion. I say that the potion will also put him to sleep, and when he wakes up, he'll become a trusting ten-year-old person. He pretends to fall asleep. He wakes up and says, "Who are you? Who are you? Where am I?"

Lailah: I like it that you didn't argue with him, not about his ludicrous demand to lock Amalia out and not about his asking you if he can go home.

Shlomo: I avoided falling into the trap of engaging in a power struggle with him, reinforcing his omnipotence defense. His parents and teachers were falling into this trap over and over again.

Anna: What did you think about his objection to his mother's not permitting him to cross the road with his scooter?

Shlomo: I thought it was good that he insisted on her treating him like a ten-year-old who can take care of his own safety. But she was right too in assessing the danger. He ignored her concern.

Ethan: He repeated the theme that had been realified by him in the previous session, that he, or the dogs representing him, had no choice but to be tough, to learn how to fight to survive. However, in the previous session he attributed the cause to his parents having been murdered. In this session the cause was his not having got enough attention from them when he was five. He still didn't trust his mother figure and saw her as bad. His proximity-control plans with respect to her were still infected with horse blinders, non-sense and fifth wheel, but these bugs began to weaken. When he said, "I'm five years old, no, ten, no, five years old". He deliberately gave you the message that he understood his confusion between the past and the present. This message attested to the weakening of his fifth wheel bug.

Daniel: You, as a magician, used suggestion. You activated the bug-buster of possible worlds to help him get rid of his fifth wheel. You also tried to make him doubt his reading of reality, busting the horse blinders and non-sense.

Anna: The whole section with the grandmother and the wolf was of course inspired by the Red Riding Hood story. When you brought in the grandmother figure,

I thought that you referred to the old woman who was his mother-substitute and died, as well as to his mother.

Shlomo: I haven't thought about it, but maybe you are right.

Good. I thought that after that session it would be advisable to invite Nadav and Amalia for a dyadic session.

Session 17.4 Nadav and Amalia

Nadav started the fifth grade.

He bursts into the apartment, angry. He tells me, "This is our last meeting!" Amalia follows, very angry. She says that Nadav has a new teacher, who called Amalia, very upset, and said that she can't handle Nadav. He walks around the classroom, disturbs the pupils, goes out of the class whenever he feels like it. If she tells him to behave himself, he refuses to listen and answers back with insolence. She is going to give up on him as a pupil.

Amalia says that he refuses to take his Ritalin, insists that it causes him nausea and stomach ache. At home he behaves the same way. He throws his clothes and socks on the floor all over the apartment, refuses to brush his teeth and take a shower. When she tells him to behave as he should, he refuses to obey and tells her to shut up. His father had decided not to intervene. Everything falls on her shoulders.

Nadav says, "I'm quitting," and runs out of the apartment. I ask her to bring him back. After five minutes she manages to get him back.

He says, "You and daddy don't love me. You've never loved me."

She says, "And who kisses you goodnight every evening?"

He says, "I don't want your kisses".

He mentions again that she forbade him to cross a road with his scooter.

She says, "If I didn't love you, I would let you cross the road and risk your life."

He says, "I want to be run over and die. I'm going to commit suicide anyway".

He lies down on the carpet, exhausted. He whispers that his parents force him to come to therapy. "It's boring here, nothing to do."

I say, "I'm bored too. I also have to force myself to come here."

He sits up and says, "Tell my mother to cut my arm." I say, "OK". I bring a large plastic knife, hand it over to Amalia and say, "Cut his arm."

She refuses to take the knife. I tell Nadav, "Shall I cut your arm?"

He says, "Yes." I pretend to cut his arm and glue a sticky red paper over the fake incision.

He says, "But you didn't really cut it."

I say, "Let's pretend that I was your mum and she really cut your arm."

Amalia does not seem to like this playful interaction. She says, "Nonsense!"

I tell her, "Don't you want to play with us?"

She says, still angry, "I don't want to play with this boy. I want him to listen to me."

He says, "I am just a boy, I'm too young to do all the things she tells me to do. It's the parents' duty, not the boy's."

I say, "Let's play as if you were a baby and Mummy changed your diaper, so your poo wouldn't get the bed dirty. Amalia, are you ready to change his diaper?"

She says, "No. He's not a baby."

He says, "Ask her if she wants to play ball with me."

She says, "I can't, I got a backache."

I ask him, "Do you care that your mother suffers from backache?"

He says, "Yes."

After a while, he adds, "I don't clean after me because I forget. If they put notes everywhere, reminding me of what I should do, I'll remember."

Lailah: He declared that he wanted to die and planned to commit suicide and she was still angry because of his disobedience and disorderliness. This unbalanced anger energized her horse blinders bug. She couldn't see his suffering, his despair, his distrust in her love, even his ADHD. She only felt her own frustration and her concern about his school performance and behavior at home. Do you think that his death wishes and threat to commit suicide were just demonstrative, or he was actually suicidal?

Shlomo: I don't know. His inner world, as portrayed in his TAT stories and play contents, was indeed haunted by demons. But it seems that in the interaction with his mother he used this threat just to frighten and punish her.

Daniel: His proximity-control plan with respect to Amalia was bugged with horse blinders and non-sense. I think his basic trust program was infected with flip-flop. He both knew and didn't know that she and his father loved him.

Ethan: I understand that you attempted to bust the bugs in Amalia's and Nadav's proximity and control plans by turning their interaction into make-believe play. When Nadav said he wanted her to cut his arm, he was trying to convey the message that he deserved to be punished for his insolence and disobedience. When you turned the cutting ritual into play, you activated owning and alienation and perhaps also arbitrariness of the signifier (a harmless piece of paper signifying blood). Also, the diapers thing. But she wasn't ready to co-operate because she was too frustrated and angry. You yourself said that the bug-busters won't work if the emotions energizing them are not re-balanced first.

Shlomo: Yes, but Nadav definitely made some progress. He, at least temporarily, suspended his omnipotence and rebelliousness and was willing to divulge to Amalia his fear that he was not a beloved son and his need to be a little boy. I think the make-believe arm-cutting helped him to own being punished for his behavior while alienating himself from the reality of the punishment. Then he offered her to reconcile, to play ball with him.

Anna: Wasn't the pretend arm-cutting too risky? I don't know if I would allow myself to touch him.

Lailah: I don't think so. It was so absurd that it could only disarm him.

Shlomo: At that point I thought that I had to convene the parents for a non-play meeting. I thought family play therapy was not going to work at that stage because of the over-loaded emotions and perhaps also because of the parents' limited insight ability.

I also asked the parents to permit me to meet Nadav's teacher and school counselor. Before I met the parents, I had another individual session with Nadav.

Session 17.5 Nadav

Nadav sits down. He says that he didn't want to come and preferred if the meeting would end. I say that I also didn't want to come, and I wanted the session to end too.

He lies on the carpet and says that he wants to sleep.

After a while he says, "I fell asleep and dreamt that I committed suicide."

He takes a toy hand-gun, aims at his temple and "shoots". He says again that he is tired and wants to sleep. He aims the gun at his stomach and "shoots" again.

I say, "And then the dream continued." I was waiting for him to tell me more. He says, "Then I dreamt that I lived on an after-death planet, where no one tells me what to do."

I say, "Let's play as if you were an astronaut and you were designed to travel to a planet where no one tells anybody what to do. I was your trainer."

He agrees. I give him instructions and he obeys.

I tell him, "Astronaut Stronghead, your three-year training program is now complete. You were our best trainee. You are now ready to go to the planet NoNoNo, where no one tells anybody what to do. Here is your spacecraft."

I give him a chair and he sits on it. I tie him with a rope and say, "During the flight you will be tied with this belt, otherwise you will float in the air and won't be able to operate the spacecraft's instruments. I'll be in the control tower and will send you instructions."

After a while I say, "Here we are, that's the planet NoNoNo! You can unbuckle your belt."

I wear a funny hat and put on gloves with long plastic nails. I say, "Let's play as if I was the king of the aliens on that planet."

I take a play slime and tell him, "I am a hospitable alien. I offer you food."

He says, "This is poison."

He takes a toy gun and "shoots" me. He says, "I killed him. Now I'm going to be the king."

I take off the hat and the gloves and say, "Earth weapons cannot kill these aliens."

He says, "Ok, so I'll stay with them and live with them."

I assume again the role of the man in the control tower and say, "Stronghead tried to kill the hospitable king of the aliens. They will turn against him and kill him. Astronaut Stronghead, you should return to earth immediately!"

He says, "No, I am staying here."

I say as the man in the control tower, "plan B! Astronaut Stronghead will be sucked into the spacecraft, which will be returned to Earth."

I add, "The space travel quickened the flow of time. When Stronghead reached the earth, he was 30 years old. He married a nice woman and had two twin children. They were a happy family and got along perfectly with each other."

Anna: I understand what you were trying to do, but I still feel worried about Nadav's suicidal ideation.

Shlomo: I was too, but I hoped that the multi-systemic therapy, which included individual, family and groups sessions, along with working with the school, remedial teaching and other types of intervention would help him be more optimistic and happier. I won't share with you the whole process, but there was considerable progress.

Daniel: You made him obey you, in make-believe. I think you activated the bug-buster possible worlds, showing him that obeying and co-operating would give him more power, not less. To be a disciplined astronaut in the training program would win him the prestige of being the first astronaut to be sent into space.

Lailah: You told him what to do in order to reach the planet where nobody tells anybody what to do. Paradox. He let you tie him. The owning and alienation let him express his weakness without giving up his omnipotence and aggression.

Shlomo: Both in the TAT stories and in the contents of his play, his suicide threats were related to the power struggles between him and Amalia, which made it impossible for both to express their love and mutual emotional dependence. It may even be that one of the motives for his opposition-defiant behavior was his unconscious fear of this emotional dependence, which could end in disappointment. The last encounter with Amalia only reinforced this emotional mess. In the next meeting with his parents, I tried to help them find a way out of this mess.

Session 17.6 Menashe and Amalia

My main purpose in this session was to help Menashe and Amalia understand the connection between Nadav's oppositional-defiant behavior and his tormented inner emotional world. Another purpose was to hold a consultation on how to obtain co-operation from him, so that he would improve his functioning on his own accord. I thought these purposes could not be achieved by family play therapy at that stage.

I shared with Menashe and Amalia the TAT results and some of the contents that came up in our play sessions. I also mentioned Nadav's declaration that he was going to commit suicide. I said that one should distinguish between his functional and behavioral difficulties, which, apparently, at least partly stemmed from his ADHD, and his emotional difficulties. They seemed to understand. Menashe himself referred to the difficult year in which the woman they lived with died and he was absent for nearly a year because of illness.

I explained to them the dysfunctional cycle of mutual frustration and anger energized by their reciprocal bugged plans for proximity and control. (I didn't use this jargon, of course.) I suggested that instead of being angry with Nadav, they could flood him with love, warmth and emotional support, but at the same time negotiate with him agreements on his rights and duties and help him implement the agreements. The expressions of love would soften him and make him more receptive and willing to co-operate.

Menashe, with his usual angry overtone, expressed doubt whether the therapy would help. He said that Nadav's real problem was his ADHD. Only Ritalin could help. He said that I analyze and dismantle the boy into parts – ADHD, learning problems, emotional problems, etc. "I am not a professional psychologist," he said, "I can only see a single entity, a whole boy who misbehaves. I refuse to tolerate his behavior, because it hurts my beloved wife, but I got tired of disciplining him. I've come to terms with the fact that Nadav is damaged and will remain damaged for the rest of his life. I'm damaged too, but I somehow manage."

I didn't try to convince Menashe that his son was not damaged, because I felt that to disagree with him would only fortify his resistance. Despite all that torrent, he said he would give the therapy a chance.

I met Nadav's teacher and the school's counsellor. I told them more or less what I said to the parents. They were very receptive. They did their best to implement my suggestions and after a while they reported a significant improvement in his behavior and functioning.

Session 17.7 Nadav, Menashe and Amalia

I convened Menashe, Amalia and Nadav for a session in which the three of them were negotiating rules of conduct at home. Nadav was disappointed, because he has looked forward to playing. I promised him to devote the second part of the session to family play, if there is time left after the conversation. But the negotiations took the whole hour.

I told Nadav that the discussion would be like in a parliament, where everyone has the right to speak. The goal will be to agree on laws and on sanctions for those who violate the laws. The parents should obey the laws too.

Nadav participated in the negotiation in a way appropriate to his age. All three of them agreed on a set of laws. Nadav asked his parents to remind him of the laws and help him keep them. He asked them again to put notes on his computer and in various parts of the apartment, as reminders.

Three days after that session Amalia called me and said that Nadav had followed most of the rules that were agreed on. She said that the atmosphere in the family improved a lot. But two days later she called me again and said that Nadav went back to his usual messy and insolent ways. He crumpled all the remaining notes and threw them at her. She and Menashe are desperate. Menashe wants to terminate the therapy because it is useless. I suggested that before declaring the therapy a failure, we hold another family meeting, try to understand what had happened and see what can be done. Amalia talked with Menashe and he consented.

Session 17.8 Nadav, Menashe and Amalia
Nadav enters the apartment alone and is sitting in front of me on the sofa in the smaller room. He says, "My father told me that when we started talking I would stop smiling."

Menashe comes in, looking belligerent, followed by Amalia, who looks extremely upset. They sit down on either side of Nadav.

Menashe says in a menacing tone of voice, glaring at me and then at Nadav, "Today I am going to do the talking."

He turns his gaze at Nadav, who refrains from looking back at him and stared at me with a frozen facial expression.

Menashe begins to speak, all a volcano of rage, "The cease-fire has ended. I'm taking over again. No parliament, no negotiations. I give orders and you obey. And if you don't, punishments. The severity of the punishment will be in proportion to the severity of the offense. At first you will not be allowed to touch your mobile phone and computer, and if you continue being messy, disobedient and insolent you will have no mobile phone or a computer. You think you are a king and we are your slaves. No, you are not a king and we are not your slaves."

Nadav, a tear crawling slowly down his cheek, is whispering, without facing Menashe, "You are adults and I'm a ten-year-old boy." He looks intimidated, not scared.

I say, "Menashe…" He turns his head at me sharply, glaring at me, and says, "No, Shlomo. You will not stop me when I'm angry!"

He continues with his diatribe, directed at Nadav, "I don't expect you to love us. I only expect you to respect us and obey us. I tear my ass off to bring bread home and you don't appreciate it. When I come back home dead tired you never ask me, 'Dad, how are you, how do you feel, how was your day?' Of course not, you don't give a damn about me or about your mother. 'Dad, did you buy me anything on your way home?' 'Dad, I'm hungry. Make me dinner.' The whole apartment looks like a garbage can and stinks, and you will never lift a finger to clean up after you. I have news for you, our apartment belongs to me, not to you."

Menashe goes on and on.

I ask Amalia, "What do you think?"

She says, "Menashe is right. I'm desperate, so I just give up and go to sleep."

Nadav looks at me and whispers, "I asked her to remind me of what I should do and to help me, but instead she kept sitting in front of the TV and watched her stupid series. I asked her to play with me with my computer game and she said it did not interest her."

To emphasize what Nadav said, I repeated and amplified it, "You asked Mommy to remind you what you should do and help you to follow the rules we had decide on, but you said that instead of reminding you and helping you she was watching her TV series that you call 'stupid' because she preferred watching instead of being with you. That's why you crumpled all the reminding notes and threw at her."

Nadav nods, affirmation.

Amalia says, "That's not how it was. I suggested that he play with me, but he preferred to be immersed in a computer game he is obsessed with all the time, so I no longer had a choice. I left him and went to watch TV."

I say, "So, he thought you preferred your series over him and you thought that he preferred his computer game over you."

Nadav says, "She always prefers her TV series. They don't love me. I know that they don't love me and they don't care about me."

Menashe says, "Are you a retard or something? We love you more than anything in the world. It is you that doesn't love us."

Nadav tells me, "Maybe they loved me a little bit when I was a baby, but then they stopped loving me. No matter what they say, I don't believe them."

All three of them fall silent, looking exhausted and deflated.

I'm trying to figure out what to say, then I say, "I'm so sad about what's happening here. The three of you suffer so much, Daddy suffers, Mummy suffers, you, Nadav, suffer. I really want to help you, but I don't know how. It would be great if you could help each other out of this mess. I have an idea, why don't we meet, all four of us, next time and instead of suffering and being so angry and upset, we'll simply play and enjoy ourselves the way we used to?"

All three of them remained silent, but I had the feeling that I had struck the right note. Indeed, they finally agreed to have a family play session.

Anna: How could you tolerate Menashe's aggression, that was directed at you and, worse, at his son. When he called Nadav "a retard" I was shocked and felt like slapping him in the face.

Shlomo: It's a kind of slang.

Anna: But did Nadav understand it that way? When his father declares that he loves him and calls him a retard?

Shlomo: Anna, you yourself said that you felt empathy toward Menashe, remember? In our discussion following the first family session, you talked about his loneliness, his desperate need for love and his deep disappointment that Nadav denies him that love. His angry outburst in the family session we are discussing now came from the same deep emotional sources.

Anna: Yes, maybe I'm ambivalent about him.

Lailah: What he said was not that extreme. It's how he said it, the unproportionate rage, that made it so intimidating.

Ethan: You made two important main moves. When you repeated and amplified what Nadav said about Amalia's failure to help him follow the rules decided on, etc., you busted the bugs horse blinders and non-sense, because you placed his relapse after the family session in the right context. I believe this message of yours registered in the minds of all three of them. The second main move was when you said that all three of them were suffering and should help each other get out of the mess. You didn't take sides. You empathized with the pain of all three of them and told them that really all three of them were on the same side and it was their mutual responsibility to solve their difficulties.

Daniel: You took a one-down position, admitted your inability to help them. I know this to be one of the kinds of strategic moves in the family therapy tradition. If you are helpless, they have no choice but to be helpful.

Lailah: Maybe the expression "get out of the mess" alluded to Nadav's being accused of making a mess and refusing to clean after himself. You conveyed the message that it wasn't only Nadav who was responsible for the mess. It was the whole family's duty to co-operate in cleaning the mess.

Shlomo: You help me understand my own moves and my own choice of expressions.

Ethan: I believe these main moves prepared the ground for Menashe to lower the level of his aggression and resistance and agree to participate in a family play therapy session.

Three days after this session Amalia called me and told me that there was an improvement in Nadav's behavior. She joined him, playing with his computer game occasionally, even though it didn't interest her at all. When she came back from work, she walked with him all over the apartment and instructed him how to collect his clothes, his socks and his notebooks, which were scattered around the floor, and how to clean up the scraps of food thrown on his desk and on the floor around it. She reminded him to wash, brush his teeth and prepare himself for sleep.

Session 17.9 Menashe, Amalia and Nadav

Nadav takes out the toy animals that participated in the family's puppet show (Observation 17.1) – the cow Moo-Moo (his own choice), the dinosaur Zaur (his father's choice) and the bear Poopy (his mother's choice). He also gets the two identical large dogs that he called the Doom Doom brothers and collects the birds of prey and the biting-stinging creatures he played with in Session 17.2.

He gives Zaur (Menashe) one of the Doom Doom brothers. He gives Poopy (Amalia) the other Doom Doom brother. He keeps Moo-Moo and the birds of prey to himself. He puts the biting-stinging creatures in Amalia's lap. Then he makes Moo-Moo and the birds of prey attack the biting-stinging creatures in Amalia's lap, in various extremely violent ways. However, he is careful not to touch Amalia herself.

I pick an owl toy and a cat toy and place them on the table above the fighting scene. I say, "The owl and the pussycat were sitting on a tree branch, watching and enjoying the battle show."

Nadav turns Moo-Moo toward the owl and the pussycat with a threatening movement, saying, "This is not a show. Go away!"

I make the pussycat ask the owl in a mewing voice, "Shall we go away? I'm afraid the cow will eat us up."

The owl says, "Don't worry, she won't. Let's stay."

Nadav continues attacking the biting-stinging creatures in Amalia's lap. He shouts, "We are killing them, they are poisonous!" He makes the birds of prey catch each of the poisonous creatures and throw it away.

Amalia says, as Poopy, "Thank you eagles, thank you Moo, you saved my life."

Menashe says, as Zaur, "Poopy, Moo-Moo didn't save your life, she saved her own life."

Nadav says, "Yes, the poisonous creatures were Poopy's army. Poopy told them to poison Moo-Moo and Doom Doom. The birds are Moo-Moo's army. Moo-Moo is their commander. Moo-Moo's army killed all Poopy's poisonous soldiers before they had a chance to kill Doom Doom and Moo-Moo."

He picks up some of the biting-stinging creatures and makes them sting some birds of prey. He cries, as Moo-Moo says, "They are back! They are back! They are poisoning my soldiers!"

He makes some birds of prey fall, one by one. The other birds of prey continue fighting with the biting-stinging creatures.

I say, as the owl, "These birds of prey are our brothers, we are all birds! They are not dead yet. Zaur, you are their brother too, because dinosaurs are the predecessors of birds! Let's help these soldiers' birds."

Menashe says, as Zaur, "They can sit on my back. I'll take them to the hospital."

Nadav says, as Moo-Moo, "No need. I have an anti-poison liquid." He pretends to cure each of the birds of prey with a liquid. They all resume the battle.

Nadav says, as Moo-Moo, "Now all the poisonous creatures are completely dead."

I make the pussycat ask the owl, "But Poopy will recruit other poisonous creatures, won't he?"

I, as the owl, answer the pussycat, "No, Moo-Moo and her soldiers cleaned Poopy's camp of any poison, forever. Poopy no longer wants to poison anybody and doesn't want any poison around him."

Amalia says, "I don't want and never wanted any poisonous creatures at all near me. I never wanted to poison Moo-Moo or Doom Doom. It was Moo-Moo who put these disgusting creatures in my lap. Maybe Moo-Moo wanted to poison me?"

Nadav says, as Moo-Moo, "No, I didn't". He takes the Doom Doom brother from Menashe's lap and makes this dog Doom Doom say, "Moo-Moo, you did try to poison Chompy, and now I'm going to kill you."

Menashe says, "Doom Doom, shut up! If you threaten Moo-Moo, I'm going to tie you on a leash and put a muzzle on your snout!"

Nadav takes Zaur and Poopy from his parents and places them on an armchair. He says, "This is the sea. Zaur and Poopy are drowning! Brothers Doom Doom, let's save them!"

He makes Moo-Moo and the Doom Doom brothers pull Zaur and Poopy out of the armchair.

I'm telling him, as the owl "They are heavy. Shall I call for help?"

He says, "No, I am stronger than them."

Immediately after he has pulled Zaur and Poopy out of the armchair, he makes Poopy and Zaur hit Moo-Moo and the Doom Doom brothers.

I say, as the pussycat, "I don't understand, why do they hit those who saved their life?"

Nadav, as Moo-Moo, "Tell the owl that they are ungrateful."

Menashe says, "Wrong! When a rescuer saves a drowning person from drowning, the drowning person sometimes panics and kicks and beats the rescuer, but not on purpose."

Nadav places Zaur and Poopy on the carpet, piles the Doom Doom brothers and all the other toys on them and lies face down on the pile with his whole body. He gets up and takes soft toys representing "nice" animals such as rabbits, puppies and hamsters out of a big box placed in the corner of the room. There are many such toys in the box. He takes out more and more, all the soft toys in the box, and places them around the pile of toys he had made before.

I say as the owl, "I think the nice animals came over to help".

Nadav takes Moo-Moo out of the pile and makes her say, "Go away, we don't need help. You are too weak to help us!" He makes Moo-Moo, The Doom Doom brothers and some of the other animals attack the nice animals and throw them away.

Then he takes Zaur and Poopy out of the pile and tells them, as Moo-Moo, "I'm going to kill you because you murdered my brothers when they were five."

I say as the owl, "I'm a thousand-years-old, so I remember that there was a war. Moo-Moo's brothers were killed by the enemies, not by Zaur and Poopy."

Nadav says as Moo-Moo, "I don't remember any war. Zaur and Poopy were the ones who murdered my brothers. I'm going to take revenge and kill them."

I say as the owl, "Moo-Moo, you lost your memory card, look here under the tree. Can you see it?"

Nadav says, as Moo-Moo, "I don't see any memory card."

I, as the pussycat, say to the owl, "Are you sure there was a war?"

I say, as the owl "O, now I remember. A part of my memory card has been erased. Zaur and Poopy took their children to the beach to have fun and told them not to go into the water alone, but they didn't listen and drowned, all of them except the Doom Doom brothers."

Nadav, as the cow says, "Zaur and Poopy were responsible. I'm going to kill them anyway."

I say, as the owl, "Don't kill them, I know someone who can download a good-parenting program and plant it in their brains."

Nadav says, "Ok, let's see if it works."

I take two play blocks and hand them over to Amalia and Menashe

I say, "You don't know me. I am the wise owl. Here are your good parenting programs. Let me plant them in your brains."

Menashe says, "We don't need any parenting programs. We are good parents. And Moo-Moo did lose her memory card. Here it is. It should be planted in her brain."

Nadav lies down on the carpet and tells Amalia to cover his whole body with pillows. The session is reaching its end.

Nadav gets out of the pile of pillows. I ask him if It felt good under the pillows. He says, "Both good and not good."

Anna: I was impressed by the co-operation of Menashe and Amalia. I thought that after the previous charged encounter, they, especially Menashe, would not agree to engage in family play therapy. All three understood the meaning of the play perfectly well and knew how to function within the make-believe world. Nadav, with all the aggression that came out of him, knew how to keep the aggression within the level of pretend. For example, he made sure not to touch Amalia physically in an aggressive way.

Lailah: I liked that you didn't immediately intervene in the play actively. Through the characters of the owl and the pussycat, you took the role of a spectator, or a participant observer. You also reframed the make-believe battle as a show that the viewers enjoy. In this way you took the sting out of the aggressive content, whether Nadav liked it or not.

Daniel: Nadav indirectly conveyed the message that his mother planned to poison him. Menashe understood this immediately – metaphorical poison.

Ethan: One of your main moves was when you said, as the owl, "Moo-Moo and her soldiers cleaned Poopy's camp of any poison, forever. Poopy no longer wants to poison anybody and doesn't want any poison in his vicinity." Through this statement, you conveyed two indirect messages. One, that it is in Nadav's power to win his mother's unconditional love and reach a peaceful and fraternal relationship with her. Two, that his mother bears no grudge against him and doesn't want to hurt him at all. In this way you tried to bust the bugs horse blinders and non-sense in Nadav proximity-control plans with respect to Amalia. You also activated possible worlds, in order to enable Nadav to imagine a relationship of harmony between Amalia and himself.

Daniel: Amalia reinforced this move by insisting that she had never wanted to poison anybody. She said that maybe Nadav was the one who wanted to poison her, and Nadav denied it.

Lailah: Another main move you made was when you enlisted Zaur's aid as someone who could help with the healing of the injured birds. You defined Zaur as a member of the poultry category and emphasized the solidarity among all types of birds. In this way, you conveyed the message that Menashe was on Nadav's side (and on your side too) and was ready to help and heal. Menashe responded well, offering to take the injured birds of prey to the hospital on his back.

Daniel: He also protected Moo-Moo against the Doom Doom brother who threatened to kill her, although he did it in his characteristic aggressive way.

Anna: Nadav refused to give up his omnipotence defense, energized by his lack of trust. He rejected any kind of help. He claimed to be able to cure the birds by his anti-poison liquid and later, when you offered help in saving the drowning Poopy and Zaur, he said he didn't need your help because he is stronger than them.

Ethan: Daniel, you mentioned Doom Doom's threat to kill Moo-Moo. Let's recall however that the purpose of this threat was to punish Moo-Moo for her intention to poison Poopy. Through the whole session, Nadav, as Moo-Moo, fluctuated between an aggressive, suspicious and blaming attitude on the one hand, and a benevolent attitude, accompanied by self-accusation, saving Poopy and Zaur from drowning, surrounding everybody with soft, nice animals, etc.; thus there were fluctuations as an emotion-balancing mechanism.

Lailah: Another main move you made was to try to get Moo-Moo to doubt her belief that Poopy and Zaur killed her brothers. I laughed when you said she'd lost her memory card.

Shlomo: As in previous sessions, Nadav was drained at the end of the session, indicating that he had done meaningful therapeutic work.

OK, the next session was with Nadav, without his parents.

Session 17.10 Nadav
Nadav brings the Doom Doom brothers, a doll representing a man and a big teddy-bear. He says, referring to the man's doll, "That's me. I am 25 years old. My name is Avi. He (the teddy-bear) was my babysitter when I was a baby. His name is Buck-Buck. He was also the babysitter of the Doom Doom brothers when they were babies".

I recall that Poopy, chosen by Amalia and representing Menashe, was a teddy-bear. I say, "Can I be Buck-Buck in the play?" He agrees.

He says, "Our uncles murdered our grandpa and our grandma and our mother and our father and tried to murder the Doom Doom brothers and me."

I say, "And Buck-Buck didn't protect you?"

He says, as the young man, "No. I killed the uncles because my saliva was poisonous. Did you collaborate with the murderers, Buck-Buck?"

I say, "God forbid! Of course not! Doom Doom brothers, Avi, do you remember me? I was your babysitter. You were so cute! I loved you so much. Can you tell me about your life since then?"

Nadav says, "All our life we've been training ourselves, and now we are so strong that no one can hurt us, and my tongue is still poisonous."

I say, "You can relax now. You are so powerful that you don't need to fortify yourselves all the time."

Nadav doesn't respond. Then he says, "Our mother and father didn't really die. They just fainted and remained fainted all those years."

I say, "Where are they? Can we wake them up?"

He says, "Here". He opens the drawer's cabinet and pulls out large dolls of a man and a woman. He lays them on the carpet. He shakes them and says, "Wake up! Wake up!" After a while he says, "They will never wake up."

I say, "They will if I sing them the lullaby I used to sing to you when you were babies."

I place the brothers Doom Doom by the man and woman dolls and start singing a lullaby, softly. Then I make the dolls wake up gradually. I stage a moving reunion, in which Nadav, as the young man Avi, gladly participates.

Ethan: I see progress. Nadav didn't regress to the critical period when he was five or six but to his infancy. The babysitter seems to be identified with his mother then. He also looked forward to his adulthood. Maybe the emotion-balancing techniques he used in the previous session and the bug-busters you activated, coupled with the basic duality of play, helped him, at least subconsciously, understand his own bugs and see his parents in a more positive light.

Daniel: He still realified the murder themes and used omnipotence as defense, but in his play his parents were no more the perpetrators, but victims, like himself. He agreed to retrieve them from their coma and participate in a moving reunion.

Anna: I liked the idea of a poisonous tongue. It is as if he is aware of his foul, aggressive language.

Lailah: You actively joined the play as the babysitter. This was a good preparatory move. As the babysitter, who was a teddy-bear like Poopy, you could put yourself in a positive, warm parental role, which was in a way a corrective emotional experience for Nadav. This role made it easier for Nadav to be receptive to your calming, encouraging messages.

Shlomo: OK, the next individual session.

Session 17.11 Nadav

Nadav suggests that we play cops and robbers. We are engaged in a shootout. He hits me, and immediately cures me with a healing ball.

I, as a cop, catch him and handcuff him with toy handcuffs. He lets me.

I take away his gun, lock him in jail and then bring him to a judge.

I tell him,"You cannot appear before the judge when you're all smeared with mud. You need a pre-shower."

He says, "I had to cover myself with mud to disguise myself, as a camouflage, so the cops wouldn't catch me, but they caught me anyway."

*Sh*lomo: Let's pretend you've already washed and the cops tell you, "Wow, I didn't know how handsome you were!"

Nadav doesn't respond, but I can see that the message has caught on.

I play the judge. I ask him why and how he became a robber. He says that both his parents were killed by robbers when he was five. The robbers raised him and taught him to be a robber.

He proposes to lead the police to the thieves who raised him. I, as a judge agree, but do not allow him to carry arms. He says the gun comes back to him as a boomerang whenever he wishes. He takes me, now as a cop, to the robbers' hideout. But then he gets the gun. He shoots me dead.

Then he turns me into the head of the band of robbers. He asks me, "How did I become a robber?" I say, your parents threw you away from home. You were homeless. We took you and made you one of us."

He says, "That's right. I was a troublemaker both at home and at school. My mum used to beat me up and I was beating her back. The robbers were smaller than me in the size of shoes and clothes."

Then he plays as if he ran away, went to the police and told them that he wants to rehabilitate and become an honest citizen. He asks them to give him an apartment in which he will raise lots of pets. He tells me, as a cop, that the robbers killed his parents. They cut an electric wire and the lamp fell on his parents and they were electrocuted.

I tell him that his parents were not killed. They only fainted. The police found them recently. They were looking for him for years.

He says, "That's not true. I left them a note, telling them that I'm with the robbers. They saw the note but didn't look for me."

I play as if I'm his parents. They told him that they regret it that they had not looked for him. They asked him to forgive them. He said, "It's too late. I don't want them to be my parents anymore."

Anna: What was the purpose of ordering him to bathe and then admiring his looks?

Shlomo: What I had in mind was the theme of people with ugly faces in his TAT stories, and also the fact that his parents kept reminding him and sometimes forced him to take a shower.

Lailah: The session gives the feeling that your rapport is getting stronger. For instance, he let you handcuff him, like when he played an astronaut (Session 17.5) and he let you tie him with a rope.

Ethan: The emotive-related realified themes are repeated here in a different disguise. He used in this session the emotion-balancing technique of fluctuations. He fluctuated, like in some previous sessions, between being the bad guy and being the good guy who repents and wants to change his ways. He also fluctuated, like in previous sessions, between the theme of being an orphan and the theme of being a bad boy who was thrown away from home.

Daniel: He had not given up on his omnipotence. The robbers who raised him were smaller than him.

Anna: You tried to bust the bug horse blinders by encouraging him to think about the causes of his oppositional-defiant behavior. "How did you become a robber?"
Shlomo: OK, let me describe a family session with Nadav, Menashe and Amalia.

Session 17.12 Nadav, Amalia and Menashe
We sit in the small room, not in the play therapy room. Nadav is disappointed. He wanted to play rather than talk. I say that we can talk and then go to the other room and play. He grudgingly consents. Amalia tells me that there has been some improvement in Nadav's behavior at home. He has been co-operative, less insolent. He demands lots of pampering gestures and hugs.

During the session, Nadav clings to Menashe, holds his hand and touches Menashe's face. Menashe hugs him but removes his hand from his face.

We go the play therapy room. Nadav hands over to Amalia the teddy-bear Poopy and to Menashe the dinosaur Zaur. He takes the cow Moo-Moo for himself and brings the brothers Doom Doom.

Nadav gets a rope and ties all the toys together. I say that the rope is not strong enough and can be easily broken. But then I pull and pull with an exaggerated effort and admit that I was wrong. The rope is very strong and cannot be broken. Nadav keeps laughing and clinging to his parents. They all hug and kiss each other and laugh.

Anna: Looks like a happy end. I like the idea of trying to disconnect the rope. A good use of the bug-buster arbitrariness of the signifier.
Shlomo: Not a happy end yet. As in every therapy, this family's idyll was not yet stable. There were ups and downs, but there is no doubt that the graph was moving upwards, in a positive direction. Let's see what the next individual session looked like.

Session 17.13 Nadav
Nadav enters the room happy, smiling and light-hearted. Throughout the session he shows his sweet side. He keeps eye contact with me and often comes physically close to me.

He piles pillows on an armchair and sits on the unstable, shaking pile.

I say, "Earthquake!" He laughs and falls to the carpet.

He says, "I died in the earthquake. Cover me with pillows, bury me."

I cover him with pillows. He says, "No, I didn't die in the earthquake. I was a robber and you were a cop and you killed me."

I say, "Your friends, the robbers, are looking for you. They are worried about you. They don't know why you didn't come back."

He sticks a finger out from under the pillows and says, "I wasn't dead, I was just unconscious for a month."

He grabs my gun and says, "I will not kill you if you give me a trillion dollars. Come with me to the ATM."

I say, "OK, but can you tell me why you became a robber?"

He says, "When I was five my parents died of a disease. No, you shot them down. They played with a toy gun and you thought it was a real gun, so you shot them. But now I want to rehabilitate. I don't want to be a robber any more. I don't like robbing and killing people. And I don't want your money. I want to recruit to the police and live on my salary."

I say, "Deep inside you are a good person."

He looks at me with appreciation and affection. For a short while he aims the gun at me and puts on a threatening expression, but immediately smiles and gives me the gun. He says, "I'll never fight again."

He lies down on the carpet and asks me to tell him a story. I start telling a story about a five-year-old boy who ... He gets up and covers my face with a pillow.

I say, "He didn't like this story."

He says, "Not in the imagination and not in real life."

Shlomo: This was followed by another family session.

Session 17.14 Nadav, Menashe and Amalia

Nadav enters the room happy, laughing, excited. Amalia and Menashe are also in a good, smiling mood.

Nadav hands over the teddy-bear to Amalia. He says, "This is little Poopy." Then he tells Menashe, "You are big Poopy." (Recall that Poopy was Menashe's nickname, given him by Amalia.)

Nadav gets many dolls, including a naked troll and puts them in Amalia's lap.

He gives some of the dolls names of popular Israeli singers. He piles pillows on an armchair and sits on the pile with each of the brothers Doom Doom by his sides.

I say, "This is King Nahadav and these are his advisors. We, his subjects, come to the palace and ask for his favors. He consults his advisors and if they recommend, he fulfills our wishes. He is a benevolent, compassionate king".

Nadav says, "But before that, they must fulfill my commandments".

I say, "And what are your commandments, His Royally?"

He says, "That little Poopy change the troll's diapers and hand him over to Big Poopy. And that Big Poopy hold all the animals in his lap."

Amalia says, "Of course, His Royally." She plays as if she changes the troll's diaper and places all the dolls in Menashe's' lap.

Menashe laughs, pets the dolls and says, "I have room on my lap for all of them."

Nadav says, "And give me all your money."

I hold the brother Doom Doom on his left and whisper in a barking voice, "His Royally, they have no money. Did you forget? All the gold in your kingdom is in the palace treasury. You are a benevolent king. You should give them money because they are poor."

Nadav says, "OK. Let them get into the treasury room and take all the gold coins that they need."

Then I tell the parents, as the Doom Doom brother, "Our king is generous, let us sing songs of praise to him. He expects it."

I was pleasantly surprised to hear both parents improvise songs of praise, as if from the mouths of the dolls representing Israeli popular singers.

Nadav lies down of the carpet and covers himself with a blanket. He says, "Now you should sing me a lullaby."

Anna: Very moving.
Lailah: He came a long way since the beginning of the therapy. Was this the last meeting?
Shlomo: No. As I said at our previous session, the therapy continued, and as expected, there were ups and downs, but the general direction was positive.

Another family session followed the last one. I asked Menashe and Amalia to bring over family photos albums. The purpose of the session was that the family tell each other their history and re-examine their respective narratives, aided by the family photos and puppets. I especially planned to concentrate on the formative years, when Nadav was five and six years old, when his father was ill and the woman who served as a substitute mother for Nadav fell ill and died. They referred to that woman as Auntie.

Session 17.15 Nadav, Menashe and Amalia

We sit in the small room. I give Menashe a Superman doll, Amalia a good-looking woman doll and Nadav a baby doll. I put aside an old woman doll, designed to represent Auntie. I hold a doll standing for a bad sorcerer in my left hand and a doll signifying a good magician in my right hand.

Nadav asks Menashe to give him the Superman doll and take the boy doll. Menashe agrees. I give Menashe a man doll.

I say, "Let's play as if the good magician has been taking care of the family and causing wonderful things to happen to it, and the evil sorcerer was jealous and has been trying to spoil things, but in the end the good magician always managed to foil the bad sorcerer's machinations."

Menashe and Amalia start to recount the history of their relationship. They role-played, through their dolls, how Menashe surprised Amalia in her workplace with a grandiose gesture of marriage proposal. He knelt down and asked for her hand, with all the employees applauding and cheering.

Nadav watches, fascinated.

Then Amalia tells how they were yearning for a child, but she couldn't get pregnant and had to go through pregnancy treatments for two years, until she succeeded in getting pregnant.

I make the good magician doll mock the evil sorcerer doll, "You see? You thought you could keep them from having a baby and being parents, but I canceled your spell."

Then Amalia tells something I didn't know, that immediately after Nadav's birth Menashe had fallen ill and had been in the hospital for two months.

Menashe, with a sad facial expression, says, "I was unlucky. I had wanted Nadav so much, I fell in love with him when he still was in Amalia's belly, but how would you say, Shlomo? The bad sorcerer did not let me enjoy my baby in the first two months of his life."

Nadav looks at Menashe, visibly moved.

I give Nadav a baby doll and say, "This was before you became a superman. Did the baby cry and missed his father?"

Nadav nods, smiling, a little embarrassed, and then makes a faint sound of a crying baby.

I make the good magician doll tell the bad sorcerer, "But after two months I won again."

Amalia shows me photos of Menashe holding the baby Nadav in his arms, his eyes sparkling with supreme love and happiness. In the other pictures it was Amalia who held Nadav, with the same euphoric facial expression. She also showed me pictures of her and Menashe embracing Nadav, both looking infinitely happy.

I show the pictures to Nadav and say, as the good magician, "Yes, I was the one who defeated the evil sorcerer."

I tell Nadav, "Let's make-believe now is then, when you were a baby and were held by Daddy and Mommy as in these photos." Nadav puts the baby doll in the lap of the man doll that's held by Menashe. The latter makes the man doll embrace the baby doll.

I say, as the good magician, "No! the real boy is now baby again. He will sit on his real dad's lap and his real dad will embrace him."

Nadav likes the idea. He quickly sits on Menashe's lap, with a big smile on his face. Menashe, embarrassed, tickles Nadav in various parts of Nadav's body. Nadav laughs and says, "I get confused, what are all those hands?"

I say, as the good magician, "The hands that dare not hug the baby."

Menashe pulls himself together and hugs Nadav in a warm embrace.

The same scene is repeated with Amalia and then with both parents holding and embracing the baby Nadav, as in the family photos.

We are reaching Nadav's fifth year. Amalia talks about Menashe's health problems, about his absence from home from almost a whole year. She says that Nadav was asking her over and over again, "Is Daddy going to die?"

I don't say anything, but show Nadav the good magician's doll.

Nadav is willing to accept the boy doll I offer him, and the doll representing Auntie. He shows how the boy and Auntie are playing all kinds of games. Then Auntie in his play is getting weaker, having difficulty getting up and walking. At this point he stops playing with the dolls and looks sad.

Amalia tells about the evening she invited a nurse to take a blood test from Auntie and the nurse came out of Auntie's room and said, "There's no one to take blood from."

Nadav says, "I knew that Auntie was dead. Mommy couldn't move and couldn't say a word. I shook her and shook her until she started crying. Daddy was at work.

Then Nadav goes on and tells, in great detail, things I had not heard before – an uncle who committed suicide, an aunt who gave birth to twins, one dead and one paralyzed.

There is a heavy silence. I walk over to Nadav, take the boy doll from his hand and give him the Superman doll. I say, "And then you became Superman."

Silence. Then Nadav is getting up, walking toward me and hitting the bad sorcerer doll with his superman doll. He says, "I killed the bad sorcerer."

Anna: Wow!
Lailah: So much illness and death Nadav experienced in his tender age of five. No wonder his stories and play were so replete with death themes. Fear of death was one of his main emotives.
Ethan: When you took the boy doll from Nadav, gave him back the Superman doll and said, "And then you became Superman," you made a move whose purpose was busting Nadav's horse blinders, by showing him the connection between his traumatic experiences and his omnipotent defense.
Shlomo: You are right.
Lailah: This therapy shows clearly the therapeutic powers of make-believe play.
Daniel: Yes, but not just make-believe play.
Shlomo: You are right. In working with the Diamond Model, play therapy is not the only method used.

Summary of chapter 17

This chapter is devoted to the presentation and discussion of the history of the case of Nadav, an oppositional-defiant ten-year-old boy, who also suffered from ADHD and an uneven cognitive profile. Play therapy was employed in individual sessions with Nadav and in family sessions. Some family sessions were dyadic – Nadav and his mother. Other family sessions included his father too. Other methods were employed alongside with play therapy, e.g. parent's guidance and consultations with the school. Nadav's behavior difficulties began in his fifth year of life. In that year a very important parental figure in his life died and his father was absent due to his health. Then, when he started school, his parents didn't understand his difficulties and were critical and angry. Nadav lost basic trust and developed an omnipotent defense. He had very pessimistic thoughts and suicidal ideations. The sessions were discussed in the interdisciplinary seminar, in which my play-therapeutic moves were analyzed and explained.

Assignments

1. Go through this chapter. Try to think of other ways in which what happened in each of the sessions can be explained. Try to think of alternative play-therapeutic moves.
2. If you are an active child therapist, try to apply the model presented in this book in your work. Analyze the cases, using the concepts, methods and techniques proposed in this book.

A classified list of publications

Play therapy with oppositional-defiant children

Bagherizadeh, H. and Nasab, H.M. (2015). The effect of play therapy on symptoms of oppositional defiant disorder in boys aged 5 to 10 years old. *International Journal of Learning & Development* 5 (2), pp.48–55.

Costello, A.H., Chengappa, K., Stokes, J.O., Tempel, A.B. and McNeil, Ch.B. (2011). Parent-child interaction therapy for oppositional behavior in children: Integration of child-directed play therapy and behavior management training for parents. In: Drewes, A.A., Bratton, S.C. and Schaefer, Ch.E. (2011). *Integrative play therapy*. Hoboken, NJ: Wiley, pp. 37–59.

Narges, N. and Babamiri, M. (2017). *Effectiveness of individual play therapy on oppositional-defiant disorder symptoms among children*. Paper presented at the 5th International Congress on Clinical and Counseling Psychology. Available at https//www.researchgate.net/publication/316804223.

Integrative play therapy

Ariel, S. (1992). *Strategic family play therapy*. Chichester: Wiley.

Ariel, S. (2002). *Children's imaginative play: A visit to Wonderland*. Westport, CT: Praeger.

Ariel, S. (2018). *Multi-dimensional therapy with families, children and adults: The Diamond Model*. London, UK: Routledge.

Drewes, A.A., Bratton, S.C. and Schaefer, Ch.E. (2011). *Integrative play therapy*. Hoboken, NJ: Wiley.

Incorporation as a defense

Hiatt, L.R. (1975). Swallowing and regurgitation in Australian myth and rite. In: Hiatt, L.R., ed. *Australian aboriginal mythology: Essays in honour of W.E.H. scanner*. Canberra: Australian Institute of Aboriginal Studies, pp.143–162.

Klein, M. (1957). Envy and gratitude. In: Klein, M. *Envy and gratitude and other works, 1946–1963*. London: Virago Press, pp.176–235.

Chapter 18

Play therapy
A reality show

Interdisciplinary seminar

Shlomo: Today I'd like us to discuss two questions: (a) How is the play therapy experience in the clinic generalized and transferred to the clients' real life? (b) How are changes achieved by play therapy in a session carried over to further sessions and accumulated in the therapeutic process?

Daniel: Do you want us to concentrate on play therapy? After all, the processes that you mentioned are affected not only by play therapy but also by other therapeutic components, and by situations and events outside of therapy.

Shlomo: You are right, of course. I'd like us to focus on the play therapy component.

Generalization and transfer from the play room to the clients' real life

Ethan: Referring to the first question, if the spontaneous play plus the play-therapeutic interventions really manage to restore emotion-balance, bust the bugs in relevant programs and promote learning and development, then the clients go home wiser, with re-balanced emotions and bug-free programs. This affects the ways they feel about and understand themselves, the others and their life. They process information differently, in more functional ways, and produce output that restores their ability to mobilized corrective feedback.

Shlomo: Can you give examples?

Ethan: Both in the first TAT story and in many sessions, Nadav (Case 17.1) reali-fied the theme of parents who died or were murdered, and left the boy an orphan, who had to be tough to survive. I think the repetition of this theme in Nadav's play had an ameliorating effect. You also helped him elaborate this theme in make-believe play. The owning and alienation and the basic duality of the play helped him gain insight into the sources of his inability to trust his parents. This weakened his horse blinders and non-sense bugs with respect to Menashe and Amalia, because he took in input and retrieved from memory information that enabled him to see his parents and his relationship with them in a different light.

In one of the sessions he played as if the dolls representing his parents would never wake up. You woke them up by singing a lullaby and staged a moving reunion. You activated possible worlds. Nadav connected emotionally to this scene. These play scenes were carried over to the real world. In the next family session, Nadav let himself seek love and warmth from his parents.

Anna: It is interesting that in the sessions that you presented to us, the theme of the ugly, deterring face that was prominent in the TAT stories didn't appear at all.

Shlomo: It did in later sessions, when Nadav was ready to delve into this sore issue.

The differential advantage of play therapy

Shlomo: What is the differential advantage of play therapy vs. verbal therapy from the viewpoint of transfer and generalization from the clinic to the real world?

Lailah: I think verbal therapy is too cognitive, too rational. The emotion-balancing powers of make-believe play and the play bug-busters bypass the defenses and create an emotional experience that also makes it possible to gain insight without going into elaborate explanations and interpretations. Make-believe play, thanks to its special nature, affects the emotions and cognitions immediately and directly, one might even say automatically.

I was impressed by the example of Tessa and her ten-year-old daughter Kate (Session 8.1). You led Tessa to be an arbitrary signifier for a hut in the forest, in which Kate found shelter. In a simple ingenious make-believe play act, you managed to expose both of them to so much suppressed cognitive and emotional information without doing any elaborate talking. The bodily and emotional experience and the symbolic meanings helped the mother and the daughter to go through a bug-busting process that was later transferred into their real life.

Failures of generalizations and transfer

Shlomo: A very good example, Lailah. I'd like to point out however that there are cases in which generalization and transfer from the play room to real life do not work.

In some cases the make-believe is taken too literally by clients, especially by adults. In other words, there is no denial of seriousness, and therefore the activity is not experienced as make-believe play. For example, a boy "kills" a doll. His parents are shocked and forbid him to play in this way.

Anna: Even if they know it's only play, they are afraid that their son is going to be a homicidal maniac.

Shlomo: Yes, but if they deny their child the playful outlet of his aggression, the moderating effect of the play will not be transferred to real life and their boy will be more likely to engage in real aggression.

Daniel: Another example would be children who play "monsters" and one of them thinks that the monsters are real.

Anna: I am thinking about the suicidal, death and murder ideations that abound in Nadav's make-believe play. Aren't all these causes of concern?

Shlomo: They are. But this is not a reason not to allow the child to realify such themes in the play. On the contrary, one should use all the heavy tools of play therapy in order to leave these contents in the make-believe realm, so that even in the real world they remain figments of the child's imagination.

Lailah: What can be the reasons for such failure?

Ethan: I can think of a number of reasons: cognitive limitations, over-heated emotions and resistance. Some children and adults are too concrete to be able to grasp the duality of make-believe play. Some children and adults are too traumatized or over-emotional to distinguish between play and reality, or to use emotional-balancing play techniques. Shlomo, you yourself told us that make-believe play can be re-traumatizing. Resistance to be playful can also be a case. For instance, at the initial stage, you preferred not to engage Menashe (Case 17.1) in family play therapy because of his resistance. The resistance can be energized by rigid defenses and inhibitions.

Daniel: From my experience, some parents, to please the family play therapist, go through the motions of make-believe play, but they are not engaged in real make-believe play, because they don't make the mental claims of realification, identification and denial of seriousness.

Anna: Can anything be done when the play therapy doesn't work?

Shlomo: There are cases in which such obstacles can be overcome. I often explain to parents why I'm doing play therapy, why it is the preferable method with little children. I tell them that when I act "silly" in the play this doesn't mean that I'm not a serious professional. With some children and their families, spontaneous, free play doesn't work, so I do structured play, such as a staged drama. I also emphasize the distinction between play and reality by means used by children, such as saying, "It's just play, it's not real"; "Now we are just making believe". I also try to create a cheerful, fun-filled atmosphere, do many preparatory and auxiliary moves before going to the main moves and provide emotional support within and outside of the play.

The therapeutic process

Shlomo: Let's move on to the second question. The therapeutic process.

Daniel: One thing I have learned from my experience is that once the therapy starts, it takes its own course. Our ability to plan the therapeutic process and predict the long-term results of our interventions is limited. Changes that have occurred as a result of carefully planned play-therapeutic moves can lead in spontaneous ways to other changes, not necessarily expected or desirable. And, on the contrary, there are cases in which our interventions do not seem to work, and we are ready to give up, and then, Oops! A fantastic breakthrough.

Shlomo: You are right. What we can do is be continuously on the alert, tracing changes within and between sessions and trying to do our best to understand their causes.

Anna: After one of the family sessions with Nadav (Session 17.12), he came to an individual session all ducky (Session 17.13). Was it a result of the family session? A culmination of all previous session? Was he just in a fleeting good mood, having a good day?

Shlomo: You are right of course, but I think the process is not that haphazard and unpredictable. Changes achieved in one session can prepare the ground for further changes, which can be reinforced by our new play-therapeutic moves. Repeating the same play over and over again in different sessions can strengthen and stabilize what has been achieved. Nadav started to exhibit guilt and self-criticism in the first sessions. These expressions were amplified in later sessions. In his play, he punished himself or asked to be punished. Later he explicitly said that he decided to change his ways.

Ethan: I think of another consideration. Since all the programs within the person and between persons are inter-related, changes that take place in one program can spread to other programs or co-occur in other programs. If Nadav (Case 17.1) is less oppositional-defiant, Menashe will be more accommodating, less critical and more optimistic about Nadav's future. Nadav's omnipotence program overlapped with his control program, in which he saw his parents as weaker than himself. If he sees his parents' strengths, he will be more likely to give up his omnipotence.

Anna: Shlomo, you seemed to like Nadav very much. I understand why. He touches a soft spot in my heart too.

Shlomo: The questions discussed in this meeting of ours are elaborated on in some of my publications, e.g. Ariel (1992).

Summary of chapter 18

In this chapter, two questions are discussed in the framework of the inter-disciplinary seminar: (a) How is the play therapy experience in the clinic generalized and transferred to the clients' real life? (b) How are changes achieved by play therapy in a session carried over to further sessions and accumulated in the therapeutic process? The main answer given to the first question was: Play-therapeutic moves that manage to restore emotion-balance, bust bugs and promote learning and development affect the ways clients feel about and understand themselves, the others and their life. They process information differently, in more functional ways, and produce output that restores their ability to mobilize corrective feedback. A question asked was what the differential advantage of play therapy vs. verbal therapy is, from the viewpoint of transfer and generalization from the clinic to the real world. It was argued that the emotion-balancing powers of make-believe play and the play bug-busters bypass the defenses and create an emotional experience that also makes it possible to gain insight, without going into elaborate explanations and interpretations. Make-believe play affects the emotions and cognitions immediately and directly, almost automatically. Another question discussed was cases in which generalization and transfer from the play room to real life do not work. In some cases there is no denial of seriousness, and therefore the activity is not experienced as make-believe play. Such failures can result from cognitive limitations, from over-heated emotions or from resistance. Make-believe play is apt to traumatize post-traumatic children. Such failures can, not in all cases, be overcome by explaining to parents the benefits of play therapy and tell them that even if the therapist acts "silly" in the play, this doesn't mean that he's not a serious professional. With resistant or less skilled clients, the play therapy can be structured rather than spontaneous. The distinction between make-believe play and non-play can be emphasized by using expressions such as saying, "It's just play, it's not real". A cheerful, festive, supportive atmosphere can be created in the room. Many preparatory and auxiliary moves can be done before going to the main moves.

As to the second question, it was pointed out that the results of play-therapeutic interventions are not always predictable. However, one should consider the following: Changes achieved in one session can prepare the ground for further changes, that can be reinforced by our new play-therapeutic moves. Repeating the same play over and over again in different sessions can strengthen and stabilize what has been achieved. Since all the programs within the person and between persons are inter-related, changes that take place in one program can spread to other programs or co-occur in other programs.

Assignments

Inspect closely the case of Nadav (17.1). Trace the processes of change within and between sessions. Try to explain the success or failure of changes to be generalized and transferred to the real, non-play world. Try to analyze and explain changes between sessions and the graph of the therapeutic process.

A classified list of publications

Change in play therapy

Ariel, S. (1992). *Strategic family play therapy*. Chichester, UK: Wiley.
Ariel, S. (2002). *Children's imaginative play: A visit to Wonderland*. Westport, CT: Praeger.
Ariel, S. (2018). *Multi-dimensional therapy with families, children and adults: The Diamond Model*. London, UK: Routledge.
Schaefer, Ch. and Drewes, A., eds. (2013). *The therapeutic powers of play: 20 core agents of change*, 2nd Edition. Hoboken, NJ: Wiley.

The play-therapeutic process

Campbell, M.M. and Knoetze, J.J. (2010). Repetitive symbolic play as a therapeutic process in child-centered play therapy. *International Journal of Play Therapy*, 19 (4), pp.222–234.

Russ, S.W. and Niec, L.N. (2011). *Play in clinical practice: Evidence-based approaches*. New York, NY: Guilford.

Chapter 19
Finale

Interdisciplinary seminar

Shlomo: This is our last meeting. I'd like us to discuss the following questions: (a) How does one know that the time is ripe for termination of an integrative play therapy? (b) What are the signs and causes of a premature termination? (c) How can one make the termination playful?

Is the time ripe for termination?

Ethan: As to the first question, I understand that you refer especially to play therapy, not to therapy at large.
Shlomo: Yes. I don't refer to a situation where it is perfectly clear that all the goals of the therapy have been achieved (although such a condition is rare and may not exist) or to the feeling of the clients that they have exhausted the therapy, but to the situation in which the individual, family or group play gives signs that the therapy is supposed to end.

Premature termination

Lailah: Isn't this related to the second question, concerning premature termination?
Shlomo: There is no straightforward way to distinguish between mature and premature termination. The feelings of both the clients and therapist that the therapy should end are very subjective and not necessarily motivated by relevant motives. I would define premature termination as cessation of therapy by the clients, which is the product of the therapist's erroneous moves, e.g. pushing the clients to change too early in the process, disregarding programs that are crucial to the therapy, lack of personal or cultural sensitivity, etc.

I almost lost Nadav (Case 17.1) when his parents allowed him to bring his smartphone to one of the sessions, and I forbade him to play with it. This was a double mistake, first because this created a conflict between the authority of his parents and my own authority, and mainly because, against my best judgment, I attempted to impose on him my own authority. That ran counter to his omnipotence defense. I had a hard time to get him back to therapy.

Termination signs in play

Anna: So what termination signs can be detected in the clients' play?

Shlomo: Many, but I'll list just a few. On the raw material level, some clients come to the meeting overdressed, as if preparing themselves for a farewell party. They keep uncharacteristic distance from the therapist, leave the room often, face outside, e.g. looking outside through the window. Or, the contrary, they approach the therapist uncharacteristically closely, touch him or her in an affectionate or aggressive way. They are overly closed or overly open physically. They are too quiet or too noisy.

Anna: This is characteristic behavior of a person who has decided to separate and leave, for instance from a partner. He finds it difficult to say so explicitly. He feels guilty or angry at himself and at his or her partner and finds it hard to take the plunge.

Lailah: Are they aware of their changed behavior?

Shlomo: Not necessarily.

On the semantic and pragmatic levels, they often avoid painful themes previously brought to light. They realify themes related to parting. They express anger at the therapist or avoid any expressions of anger. They are unusually sad or unusually cheerful. They express over-appreciation of the therapist or, the contrary, devalue his contribution.

Daniel: I have witnessed such behaviors in my practice. Separation is never easy, even if it is the right and necessary thing to do.

Playing the final notes

Ethan: You mentioned playful termination. I sometimes encourage termination even if the clients are reluctant to end the therapy. They are likely to feel rejected. Then I try to help them express their anger and sadness in make-believe play.

Shlomo: Another technique I use is encouraging make-believe play regression, summarizing the history of the therapy in make-believe, play a make-believe continuation of the therapy and play with the clients a possible future world.

Since this is our last meeting, I suggest that we now do a make-believe play termination and see how it works.

Anna: An excellent idea.

Anna, Ethan, Daniel, Lailah and I start enthusiastically to engage in a make-believe play farewell party.

Summary of chapter 19

In this chapter, questions concerning the termination of an integrative play therapy are discussed. The questions are (a) how does one know that the time is ripe for termination of an integrative play therapy? (b) What are the signs and causes of a premature termination? (c) How can one facilitate the termination by making it playful? It is said that it is not easy to distinguish between timely and premature termination. The latter can be defined as a decision of clients to leave because of an erroneous move done by the therapist. It is stated that there are signs of approaching termination in the clients' play behavior, both when the termination is timely and when it is premature. The signs are manifest in the clients' play behavior on the raw-material, semantic and pragmatic levels, especially if the clients find it difficult to explicitly express their wish to terminate. Separation is never easy, even if it is unavoidable. It involves feelings of guilt, anger and sadness. The participants suggested make-believe play techniques designed to facilitate the separation.

Assignments

1. Describe your own feelings and behavior when you part with an important person in your life.
2. If you are an experienced therapist, describe your behavior and the clients' behavior in the stage of terminations.
3. Suggest more termination play techniques.

A classified list of publications

Premature termination

Ariel, S. (2018). *Multi-dimensional therapy with families, children and adults: The Diamond Model*. London, UK: Routledge.

Midgley, N. and Navridi, E. (2007). An exploratory study of premature termination in child analysis. *Journal of Infant, Child and Adolescent Psychotherapy*, 5 (4), pp.437–458.

Swift, J. K. and Greenberg, R.P. (2015). *Premature termination in psychotherapy: Strategies for engaging clients and improving outcomes*. Washington, DC: American Psychological Association.

Termination in play therapy

Ariel, S. (1992). *Strategic family play therapy*. Chichester, UK: Wiley.

Kranz, P.L. and Lund, N.L. (1979). A dilemma of play therapy termination anxiety in the therapist. *Teaching* 6 (2), pp.108–110.

List of cases, sessions and observations

Cases

1.1 Rusella
3.1 Max
3.2 Kabr
10.1 Shan
11.1 Bella
11.2 Erez
11.3 Meera
13.1 Gad
13.2 Bassel
16.1 Lucy
17.1 Nadav

Sessions

1.1 Lailah and Rusella
8.1 Tessa and Kate
8.2 Sofia
9.1 Eli and his mother
9.2 Daliah
9.3 Ashley
11.1 Rex
15.1 Gad
15.1 (2) Gad, contd
15.1 (3) Gad, contd
15.2 Gad, Benny and Esther
15.3 Group play therapy with Gad
17.1 Nadav
17.2 Nadav
17.3 Nadav
17.4 Nadav and Amalia

17.5 Nadav
17.6 Menashe and Amalia
17.7 Nadav, Menashe and Amalia
17.8 Nadav, Menashe and Amalia
17.9 Menashe, Amalia and Nadav
17.10 Nadav
17.11 Nadav
17.12 Nadav, Amalia and Menashe
17.13 Nadav
17.14 Nadav, Menashe and Amalia
17.15 Nadav, Menashe and Amalia

Observations

5.1 Ava and grace
5.2 Shay and Gal
6.1 Tamar
6.2 Tamar
6.3 Jonathan
7.1 Easy riders
7.2 Sara, Gabby and Maayan
9.1 Eric and Alina
9.2 The power of good and the power of evil
10.1 Motor development – balance
10.2 Attention and perception
10.3 Creative thinking and problem-solving
10.4 Memory, planning and organization
10.5 Self and body images and concepts
10.6 Self and body boundaries
10.7 Empathy and pro-social attitude
10.8 Self-control and postponing gratification
11.1 Lee
11.2 Rana
11.3 John and Leo
11.4 Paul
11.5 Ian
13.1 A family free play session
16.1 Maya and Lucy
17.1 Nadav, Menashe and Amalia

Index

abreaction 5, 111
arbitrariness of the signifier as a play bug-buster 71, 75–77, 83, 109, 154, 174, 209; *see also* bug-busters
associative thinking 109
attachment 19, 83, 112, 167; disorder of 6

basic duality, as a play bug-buster 70, 77, 83, 94, 109, 179, 199, 207; *see also* bug-busters
body, as a subsystem; *see also* subsystems
bug-busters 24–25, 28, 70, 83, 109, 119, 184, 190, 194, 199, 201, 207, 209; play bug-busters 28, 70, 83, 109, 119, 184, 190, 194, 199, 201, 207, 209; *see also* bugs in information-processing programs
bugs in information-processing programs 23–24, 92, 119, 157, 179, 184, 186, 191, 194, 199

Carnap, Rudolf 12
catharsis 5, 111; *see also* therapeutic powers of play
change mechanisms, types of 25
child-centered play therapy 1
cognitive and psychomotor subsystems 19, 20; *see also* subsystems
comprehensiveness, as a property of simplicity 22, 28, 184; *see also* simplicity, as a central explanatory principle
concretization, as a type of change mechanism 25; *see also* change mechanisms, types of
consistency, as a property of simplicity 22, 28, 180–181, 184; *see also* simplicity, as a central explanatory principle

Context-Dependent Componential Analysis 47–54, 131; as a map of a cybernetic emotion-balance mechanism 50; as a dictionary of the players' private contents 50, 131; *see also* cybernetics; emotion-balancing
counter-conditioning 111
counter-transference 9
creativity 112
crisis and change 23
culture, internalized 19; *see also* subsystems
cybernetics 21, 22, 119, 123

deep structure 42
denial of seriousness 110; *see also* make-believe play
development, dimensions of 20, 28–29, 88–94, 123–136, 160, 169; of attention and perception 89; of creative thinking and problem-solving 89; of empathy 90; of memory, planning and organization 89; of motor development 88; of self and body boundaries 90, 160, 169; of self and body images and concepts 90; of self-control, 91
developmental profiles 2, 20, 123, 124–136
Diamond Model, The 1, 19–29; reasons why developed 19
distancing, as an emotion-balancing device 100–101; *see also* emotions, as a subsystem; emotion-balancing; emotive
dreams, compared to play 109, 110

ecology 5, 20
egocentricity 19; *see also* development, dimensions of

emotion-balancing 103–104, 111, 130, 149, 154, 159, 167, 171, 179, 184, 188–189, 199, 200, 207, 209; compared to defense mechanisms 103; *see also* emotive
emotions, as a subsystem 19, 92, 96–104, 111; as a cybernetic cognitive-affective mechanism, 96–99; positive 111; unbalanced 92, 96–104; *see also* emotion-balancing; emotive
emotive 49, 54, 96–98, 110, 124, 130, 165, 167–169, 171, 181–182, 200; core and periphery of 110, 124, 165, 181–182, 200; as an emotional-balancing mechanism 95–98, 110, 124, 130, 165, 167–169, 171, 181–182, 200; sensitizing cognitive processes 97; *see also* emotions, as a subsystem; emotion-balancing
empathy 19, 112
empowering and immunization 101 *see also* therapeutic powers of play
enhancing alertness, as a type of change mechanism 25; *see also* change mechanisms, types of
explicating, as a play-therapeutic technique 148; *see also* moves, play-therapeutic; play-therapeutic session, structure of
explication, Carnap's concept of 12, 6, 67–68; of the concept of make-believe play 12, 67–68; *see also* Carnap, Rudolf; make-believe play
expression and catharsis, as a type of change mechanism 25; *see also* change mechanisms, types of

family play therapy 1, 142, 154–157, 173–175, 177–181, 187–198, 201–205
family systems 20
feedback, corrective 21; *see also* cybernetics
feed-forward 21; *see also* cybernetics
fifth wheel, as a bug 23, 77, 180, 186 *see also* bugs in information-processing programs
flip-flop, as a bug 23, 76, 82, 125, 184; *see also* bugs in information-processing programs
focusing, as a play-therapeutic technique 148; *see also* play-therapeutic session, structure of

generalization and transfer 207–209, failure of 208–209; overcoming such failures 209; *see also* play therapy
genetics 5; *see also* development, dimensions of
group play therapy 142, 157–161

habituation, as a type of change mechanism 5, 25; *see also* change mechanisms, types of
homeostasis 21; *see also* cybernetics
horse blinders, as a bug 23, 77, 82, 123, 125, 160, 169, 180, 186, 188, 194, 201, 205; *see also* bugs in information-processing programs

identication, as a part of the definition of make-believe play 110; *see also* make-believe play
idiographic theory 22, 50
illusion of alternatives 148, 160; *see also* moves, play-therapeutic
individual play therapy 142–143, 149–154, 165–167, 170–172, 181–187, 189–190, 198–202
influence and suggestion, as a type of change mechanism 25; *see also* change mechanisms, types of
influencing information-processing, as a type of change mechanism 25; *see also* change mechanisms, types of
information-processing 21, 25, 119; *see also* Diamond Model, The
interpretation 6
introducing protective devices or curing agents 101; *see also* emotion-balancing

joining the clients' play 2, 150; *see also* moves, play-therapeutic

language, theoretical, of the Diamond Model 21–22
life events 5, 20; *see also* subsystems
linguistic peculiarities of make-believe play 81–86, 150, 154, 159; *see also* make-believe play

macroscopic analysis 42, 47–54, 56–63; on the pragmatic level 56–63; on the semantic level 47–54
make-believe play 1, 6, 13, 15, 37, 42–44, 47, 67–70, 81–86, 88–94, 96–104,

109–110, 150, 154, 159, 205–207; ambiguity of expressions of time and place in 82, 83; as bug-busters 81–86, 205; compared with dreams 109, 110; definition of 13, 67–68; differences from akin phenomena 68–70, 207; as an emotion-balancing mechanism 96–104; linguistic peculiarities of 81–86, 150, 154, 159; meta-cognition in 15, 81; misconceptions about 15; recording and analyzing of 1, 37, 42–44, 47; use of past tense in 85; as a vehicle of learning and development 88–94, 159; verbal and non-verbal aspects of 15; *see also* bug-busters; emotion-balancing; linguistic peculiarities of make-believe play; meta cognition; recording techniques of observed play; semiotic analysis of play

meta-cognition 15, 81, 85

microscopic analysis 42; *see also* semiotic analysis of play

mimicking 147; *see also* play-therapeutic session, structure of

miniaturing 111

monitoring the play-therapeutic process 2, 209–210; *see also* play-therapeutic process

moral development 19, 112; *see also* developmental dimensions

moves, play-therapeutic 147, 159, 160, 194, 197, 198, 199, 205; *see also* play-therapeutic session, structure of; play therapy

multi-systemic 1, 2, 19, 119–136, 143, 178, 190; diagnostic profile 2, 119–136; as a property of The Diamond Model 19, 178, 190; *see also* Diamond Model, The

neutralizing 101; *see also* emotion-balancing

non-sense, as a bug 23, 76, 169, 180, 186, 194; *see also* bugs in information-processing

obedient actor 149; *see also* moves, play-therapeutic; play-therapeutic session, structure of

object relations 19

observation techniques, of play 37–39; common observation errors 37

obsessive-compulsive disorder 5

owning and alienation, as a play bug-buster 70, 75, 77, 109, 169, 174, 179, 207; *see also* bug busters

pacing 147; *see also* moves, play-therapeutic; play-therapeutic session, structure of

parsimony, as a property of simplicity 22, 27, 184; *see also* simplicity, as a central explanatory principle

personality, as a subsystem 19; *see also* development, dimensions of

planning a play-therapeutic session 2; *see also* strategy, play-therapeutic

plausibility, as a property of simplicity 22, 27, 180, 184; *see also* simplicity, as a central explanatory principle

play 2, 12–15, 25, 108–113; no single definition of 12, 13; as a semiotic system 14–15; therapeutic powers of 2, 25, 108–113; *see also* make-believe play; therapeutic powers of play

play-therapeutic process 2, 209–210

play-therapeutic session, structure of 147–149

play therapist, roles of 6, 147; *see also* play therapy

play therapy 5–6, 12, 14, 16, 74, 150, 153, 209; advantages of 209; being re-traumatized by 14; child-centered 6; cognitive-behavioral 5; concept of 14; current state of 12; dangers of 14; directive, 14, 74, 150, 153; dynamic 5; evidence-based 5; flexibility of 6; integration of models of 12, 16; models of 12; requirements of a model of 14; target-oriented 5; wealth of therapeutic means of 6; *see also* play-therapeutic process; play therapy session, structure of

positive reinforcement and support, as a type of change mechanism 25; *see also* change mechanisms, types of

possible worlds as a play bug-buster 71, 77, 109, 169, 190, 208; *see also* bug-busters

pragmatic level of semiotic analysis 42; *see also* semiotic analysis of play; semiotics

presenting problems 5

presuppositions of a structure 44; *see also* pragmatic level of semiotic analysis programs, information-processing 23; *see also* simplicity as a central explanatory principle

providing stimuli 148; *see also* moves, play-therapeutic; play-therapeutic session, structure of

proximity and control 27, 44, 57–63, 92, 123–136, 165–169, 175; 180, 186, 191, 194, 197; goals and plans of 57–63, 123–136, 165–166, 167–169, 175; metaphorical images of 57–63; purposes and presuppositions of 44; tactical mean of 57–63; *see also* semiotic analysis of play

psychosexual development 19; *see also* development, dimensions of

psychotherapy integration 16; *see also* Diamond Model, The

purpose of a structure 44; *see also* pragmatic level of semiotic analysis

raw material of observed behavior 37, 42; *see also* semiotic analysis of play

realification 13, 67–68; *see also* make-believe play

reality testing 19; *see also* development, dimensions of

recording techniques of observe play 37; *see also* observation techniques, of play

repetition in a safe environment 99, 100; *see also* emotion-balancing; moves, play-therapeutic; play-therapeutic session, structure of

resiliency 111

resistance 142

reversing 102; *see also* emotion-balancing; moves, play-therapeutic; play-therapeutic session, structure of

self and body, image and concept 19, 90; boundaries of 19, 90; *see also* development, dimensions of

self-esteem 113; *see also* development, dimensions of

self-control 19, 91, 113; *see also* development, dimensions of

semantic level of semiotic analysis 42–44, 47–54; *see also* semiotic analysis of play

semiotic analysis of play 15, 42–44, 47; pragmatic level of 42–44, 47; raw material level of 42; semantic level of 42; therapeutic benefits of 15, 42

semiotics 1, 2, 21 42–44, 47–54; *see also* semiotic analysis of play

simplicity, as a central explanatory principle 22–29, 123–126, 130–136, 180, 184; aspect of 28; attempts to restore partially 24, 123, 125, 130–136, 180, 184; loss of 24, 26–29, 123–126; *see also* bugs in information-processing programs

social competence 112

social systems 20; *see also* multi-systemic

stopping 102 *see also* emotional-balancing mechanisms

strategy, of play therapy 2, 140–143, 169–170; components of 141, 169–170

structures, as sequences of raw-material-semantic units 43–44, 57–63, 132–136; *see also* semiotic analysis of play

subsystems 19–20, 123–124; external, 19, 20, 123–124; internal, 19, 20; *see also* multi-systemic

surface structure 46

symbols, as taken from an emotive's periphery 110; *see also* emotives; emotional-balancing mechanisms

synchronic vs. diachronic perspectives 88, 119, 122

technical eclecticism 25

termination 2, 213–214; play techniques for 214; premature 213; signs in play 214

the double 148; *see also* moves, play-therapeutic

therapeutic powers of play 2, 109–113; *see also* make-believe play

transitions in a play therapy session 9

trauma 26, 130

unconscious, access to through play 109, 110, 119

ups and downs 100; *see also* emotion-balancing

willy-nilly 149; *see also* moves, play-therapeutic

working through the body, as a type of change mechanism 25; *see also* change mechanisms, types of

THE ENGLISH CIVIL WAR Around Wigan and Leigh

by
Fred Holcroft

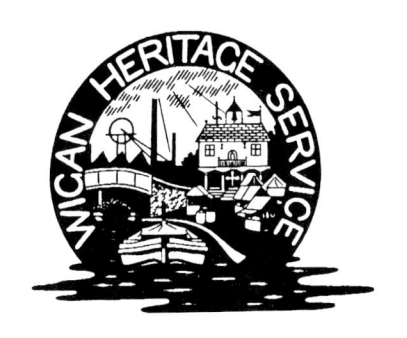

First published August 1993
by
Wigan Heritage Service
Leisure Services Dept.
Wigan MBC
Market Suite
The Galleries
Wigan WN1 1PX.

No part of this book may be reproduced, stored in a retrieval system, or transmitted in any form, or by any means, electronic, mechanical, photocopying, recording, or otherwise, without the prior permission of Wigan Heritage Service.

© Wigan Heritage Service, 1993.

ISBN 1 874496 03 X

Designed and produced by Coveropen Ltd., Wigan.
Tel: (0942) 821831

Contents

Chapter 1
The Drift to War 5

Chapter 2
War Begins 9

Chapter 3
Ebb and Flow 11

Chapter 4
Breakthrough 17

Chapter 5
Prince Rupert 21

Chapter 6
Oliver Cromwell 26

Chapter 7
The Battle of Wigan Lane 30

Chapter 8
Aftermath........................ 34

Chapter 9
Conclusion 38

To Mr. P. W. Skirrow,
former history master at Wigan Grammar School.

Chapter 1

The Drift to War 1628-1641

IN many ways conditions in early 17th century Lancashire reflected those in the country at large: conflicts caused by religion, political ambition, economic change and a hostility to the personal government and personality of King Charles I. Events in Wigan from the very beginning of Charles I's reign illustrate this. In the Parliamentary election of 1628 the result was:

    Sir Anthony St. John   (65 votes)
    Edward Bridgeman   (63 votes)

Wigan was entitled to two M.P.s; in this case both those elected were Royalist sympathisers and while Bridgeman was a Protestant, St. John's Roman Catholic faith did not prevent him from topping the poll. Two further candidates held Royalist sympathies but the most remarkable feature of the occasion was the attempt by three Wigan craftsmen to get themselves elected. The Mayor would not allow anyone who was not a burgess of Wigan to vote and the gentry and burgesses ensured the victory of their candidates. Peter Houlford who came joint fourth in the election was a journeyman craftsman and probably the first 'labour' candidate at a Parliamentary election anywhere.

During the years that followed, King Charles I increasingly alienated his subjects, even those in a town as loyal as Wigan. First he dissolved Parliament and ruled England alone for 11 years. During this period of personal rule his main problem was raising the money to run the country and this is where Charles really lost friends and made enemies. One of the taxes over which he still had control was the raising of Ship Money. This was an accepted measure in wartime but its peacetime use as an excuse for bringing in money was resented everywhere and became a focal point for resistance. In 1634 Lancashire was rated at one ship of 400 tons, costing £1,000. This was divided between the various towns and villages in proportion to their relative wealth and importance and at the top of the list were:

Wigan £50
Preston £40
Lancaster £30
Liverpool £25

At the election in April 1640, for what later became known as the Short Parliament, the political climate was very different. There were six candidates, four Royalists (two Protestants and two Roman Catholics) and two Parliamentarians. Elected were:

Orlando Bridgeman (112 votes)
Alexander Rigby (104 votes)

The most startling change was that Sir Anthony St. John, who had headed the poll in 1628, came next to the bottom with only four votes. His fellow Roman Catholic candidate got only one. This time Wigan had elected two very different members, destined to become famous on opposite sides in the Civil War. Orlando Bridgeman, son of the Rector of Wigan, a Protestant and a keen Royalist, topped the poll while Alexander Rigby, a staunch Puritan and opponent of the King came a close second. Once again the Mayor would not allow non-burgesses to vote, despite their protests.

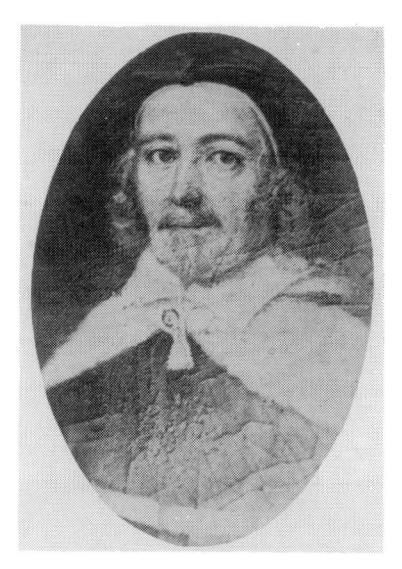

Alexander Rigby, M.P. for Wigan in the Parliamentary Cause 1640-1650, and Colonel in the Parliamentary Army.

For a second time Charles dissolved Parliament when he found he could not get his own way, but was forced to call another election six months later in October 1640. This time there was pandemonium at the Wigan polling booths. In those days there was no such thing as a secret ballot. On the day of the election, everyone gathered at the Moot Hall—candidates, voters and anyone else who cared to turn up. The names on the voters' list were called out by the clerk and as each man indicated his choice the candidates's name was written against that voter's name in the poll book, which has been preserved for posterity. Once everyone had chosen, but before the Mayor was able to declare the result, those who had not been allowed to take part in the election began to shout and demonstrate, demanding to be allowed to vote. No document survives indicating who they wanted to support, but the Mayor felt it necessary to write to the Speaker of the House of Commons asking him to uphold the Mayor's decision to once again exclude the non-burgesses. Although the Speaker backed the Mayor the townsmen were not satisfied and in the weeks that followed there were public meetings, demonstrations and demands for a new election. The distribution of votes in the October 1640 election shows just how opinion had hardened against the King. Rigby the Parliamentarian this time headed the poll with 136 votes against 128 for the Royalist Bridgeman. Robert Gardner, Bridgeman's fellow Royalist candidate who had received 72 votes in April, this time received only 57.

In this part of the county the Royalist cause came to be inspired and dominated by one man — James Stanley, Lord Strange. Aged 35 when war broke out in 1642 he was soon to inherit his father's title of Earl of Derby.

Strange had always been on good terms with his neighbours, and although himself a strong Anglican, as the leading local magistrate he had dealt leniently with both local recusants and Protestant dissenters. A moderate, he had tried to arrange a compromise between the two sides in Lancashire. Some Parliamentarians had hoped that Strange would be their leader and had conducted secret negotiations with him.

One of the largest landowners in the region, the Derby family dominated west Lancashire from their seat, Lathom House near Ormskirk. When war broke out the Royalists were able to hold the coastal lowland areas for the King, as far west as Warrington, Preston and Wigan. By contrast the eastern part of the county, the Hundreds of Blackburn and Salford, were held for Parliament. Wigan therefore found itself from the start in the front line.

Wigan in 1640 was a prominent market town on a low hill partly protected by the River Douglas and overlooking the river for some miles. The Market place in the town centre contained the church, the Moot Hall, inns, shops and houses of the more wealthy inhabitants. It must have been a picturesque sight — buildings built of timber and clay, with overhanging first floor rooms and thatched or flagged roofs. From the Market Place opened the four main streets, Standishgate, Millgate, Hallgate and Wallgate. Strategically Wigan straddled the main north-south highway and guarded the crossings of the Douglas. Some of the local industries, such as metal-working, could be adapted for the manufacture of weapons. A Royalist writer noted that Wigan was:

> "much in favour of the Earle, a town which he had confidence in above any other in the county".

Supporters of Parliament were not so complimentary. One wrote that Wigan was:

> "such a malignant towne as the like was not in all the county".

Wigan later came to the notice of the great Oliver Cromwell himself who looked on it as:

> "very malignant".

Throughout 1641 the country drifted towards war and small incidents recorded in Wigan show what was happening. In March some of William Wood's neighbours complained of his beating a drum in the middle of the night; he defended himself by explaining that he had been ordered to do it:

> "to call my fellow soldiers together being warned to be at Ormskirk by eight of the clock on pain of death".(1)

The town bailiffs were ordered to make butts for target practice and two men, William Harvey and Ralph Holland, were admitted as tradesmen in the town so that they could manufacture:

> "bills and other warlike weapons for the safeguard of the town in any time of danger".(2)

Another tradesman, Richard Gregson, enquired that

> "being informed that your towne of Wigan hath need of a gunn smith"(3)

applied for the post and was taken on. Geoffrey Scott, a noted Wigan bellfounder, made a "brake gun" (a type of cannon) which was mounted on the town walls.

The other side was also preparing for war and a Puritan could proudly write:

> "we are all about our guard and the naylers [nailmakers] of Chowbent [Atherton], instead of making nayles, have busied themselves in making bills and battle axes."(4)

To the ordinary people as well as those in high places it looked as if war was inevitable.

Chapter 2

War Begins

BY the spring of 1642 King and Parliament had come to the conclusion that war was indeed inevitable. Charles I left London on 10 January 1642 and he was never to return except as a prisoner. On 10 March 1642 he met at York with his chief northern supporters, including Lord Strange, who was there to represent his dying father. Charles issued commissions of array authorising them to raise troops on his behalf. Strange returned to Lancashire and began to arm his own tenants and to recruit his friends and neighbours. Parliament countered by appointing Lord Wharton as its Lord-Lieutenant of Lancashire, and he soon succeeded in organising those gentry prepared to actively oppose the King. Many, however, remained neutral. Clarendon, the King's own historian, was forced to write:

> "many thought that they had done enough for the King in that they had done nothing against him".

The first trial of strength in Lancashire between the two sides took place on open ground just outside Preston on 20 June 1642. Lord Strange had called a meeting of his supporters in accordance with instructions from the King. Hearing of his intention, Alexander Rigby, MP for Wigan, and Richard Shuttleworth, MP for Preston, rode north to prevent as many people obeying the summons as possible. At Standish they deprived the Constable of his warrant and at the Preston site they warned those assembled that the proclamation was not sanctioned by Parliament and therefore unlawful. The meeting was plunged into confusion as several thousand armed men milled about. The meeting broke up in turmoil but without bloodshed.

On 15 July 1642 an extraordinary incident occurred. The many Royalist sympathisers still inside Manchester invited Lord Strange to a dinner in the town at the house of Alexander Green. There was a scuffle and a shot rang out. One of Strange's party had shot and killed Richard Percival a linen webster. This is thought to have been the first casualty of the English Civil War anywhere in the country.

In August 1642 King Charles raised his standard at Nottingham and called on all his loyal subjects to rally to his cause. Lord Strange was impeached by Parliament for his part in the Manchester affray. The Civil War had begun.

Strange decided to strike the first blow and on Saturday 24 September 1642 he again arrived at Manchester, this time with a large force variously estimated at between 2,000 and 4,500 men with seven cannons. A meeting of Manchester's inhabitants had put the militia on a war footing, raised an extra regiment of foot under the command of Richard Holland of Denton, and with this force taken possession of Manchester in the name of Parliament. Being short of military experience they had hired a German mercenary soldier and military engineer, John Rosworm, who had fought on the Continent during the Thirty Years' War and in Ireland against the Roman Catholic rebels. Since Strange's last visit the town had been fortified by Rosworm and Holland against a sudden attack. The town was full of armed men headed by most of Parliament's local leaders. Throughout the week-long siege the defenders received encouragement from their clergy, who visited the men at their posts. Regular prayer meetings and psalm singing, even in the ale houses and taverns, kept spirits high. Probably just as important an obstacle to Strange was the Manchester rain which fell incessantly all week, dampening the enthusiasm of the besiegers in their makeshift quarters. Against such a resolute defence Strange had no success. He tried to extract some demands from the defenders but without effect. Further disheartened by the news that his father had died, Strange gave up all hope of taking Manchester by a direct assault. On 1 October 1642 he marched away with all his forces and his new title of Earl of Derby. Manchester had been saved for Parliament.

Chapter 3

Ebb and Flow

THE Earl of Derby did not know it at the time but his repulse at Manchester signalled the defeat of his whole enterprise, and within seven months the Royalists had lost control of this small theatre of operations. But before then the war ebbed and flowed across the county in an almost bewildering pattern.

During October and November 1642 the Earl raised and equipped forces in Lancashire and sent them to join the main Royalist army at Shrewsbury. A short time later he made Wigan his headquarters.

Both sides sent out raiding parties and on Sunday 27 November 1642 a Royalist cavalry patrol was spotted approaching Chowbent (Atherton). The alarm was raised and a scratch force of both cavalry and infantry, but consisting mainly of inexperienced civilians, assembled. The Royalists, hopelessly outnumbered, made a fighting retreat through Leigh to

MAP 1 : EBB AND FLOW : September - December 1642

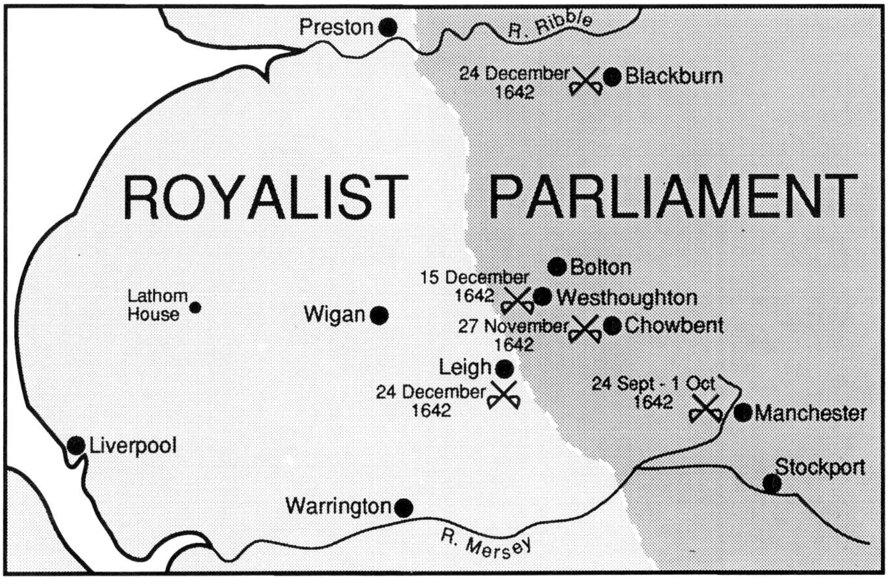

Lowton, chased by the enthusiastic Parliamentarian cavalry who left their infantry behind struggling to catch up. Turning on their pursuers the Royalists counter-attacked but in a short sharp skirmish were beaten and rode off, leaving behind almost 200 prisoners and some dead and wounded.

On 10 December 1642 the Royalists held a meeting in Preston, called for the purpose of:

> "recruiting the king's forces and raising the necessary supplies for their support".(5)

It was resolved that 2,000 foot (infantry) and 400 horse (cavalry) should be recruited and the sum of £8,700 levied on the county for their supplies. These troops were only to be used for the defence of Lancashire. The same meeting fixed the daily rate of pay for the soldiers as:

Foot	s	d	Horse	s	d	Dragoons	s	d
Captain	10	0	Captain	10	0	Captain	12	0
Lieutenant	4	0	Lieutenant	8	0	Lieutenant	6	0
Ancient	3	0	Cornet	6	0	Cornet	4	0
Sergeant	1	6	Corporal	4	0	Sergeant	3	0
Drummer	1	3	Trumpeter	3	0	Kettle Drum	2	0
Corporal	1	0	Private	2	0	Corporal	2	0
Private	0	9				Private	1	6

A few days later on 15 December 1642 the Royalists had their revenge for their defeat at Leigh when they surrounded a Parliamentarian force at Westhoughton, compelling them to surrender. On Christmas Eve, however, a Parliamentarian force took Leigh (which had been re-occupied by the Royalists) with the loss of only one man. On the same day Royalist Sir Gilbert Hoghton made a half-hearted attempt to take Blackburn but was beaten off, the attackers retreating under cover of darkness after a desultory bombardment which did negligible damage. A contemporary Parliamentary pamphleteer put it contemptuously:

> "upon Christmas day at night, Sir Gilbert withdrew his forces, being weary of his siege and his soldiers and clubmen were glad of it that they might eate their Christmas pyes at home. But they did the good man about whose house they lay, much harm, not only in eating his provision of meale and beef and the like as also in burning his barn doors with his carte wheels and other husbandry stuff."

After these early skirmishes military etiquette was brought into action as both sides exchanged prisoners. On the Royalist side, Hugh Anderton of Euxton was responsible for the exchange of prisoners. His papers are preserved in the Wigan Archives. Among them are documents giving information about casualties at the various encounters. Different types of soldiers had different values put on them. One note says:

> "Abraham Hilton
> Anthony Cocke
> John Ogden   3 drummers for 6 common soldiers.
> The rest may be exchanged for men of the like qualitie."(6)

And another one adds:

> "Israell Edge For
> John Marsh
> John Ogden
> Abraham Hulton
> Anthony Cocke."(7)

As might be expected with such complicated methods of negotiation, mistakes were sometimes made:

> "you have sent me one short of the number I sent you, the messenger lost your list, I pray send me one to supply his defect."(8)

Similarly:

> "we are mistaken in sending Robert Caterall in the supply of the 57 names. I have therefore sent you in this paper the name of an other souldier in stand of his viz Edward Butcher of Rainforth listed under Captain Marshall."(9)

Sometimes the soldiers themselves took advantage of the system:

> "Fletcher who was sent with Captain Browne to Bolton I hear since the writing of my last letter is with his wife in Prestwich parish it seems he is a knave, I pray be pleased to release the messenger you have at Wigan detained for him and use your best means to plague the man who hath dealt falsly with you."(10)

Often a little pleading or some moral blackmail had to be employed:

> "Sir I will not write a falsity I pray consider James Holden is a very poore man hath a wyfe and 10 children."(11)

And another pathetic note:

> "these whose names are within written have hitherto been maintained by my Lord of Derby his charity and are many of them wounded men I desire and expect they should be first exchanged. They being all at Wigan and now lie in the most sufferance."(12)

There were always those caught up in the fighting through no fault of their own. At the bottom of a long list of Parliamentary prisoners who had been captured at Westhoughton on 15 December 1642 is the name and comment:

> "Robert Miller of Manchester carrier of the magazine prest for that service".(13)

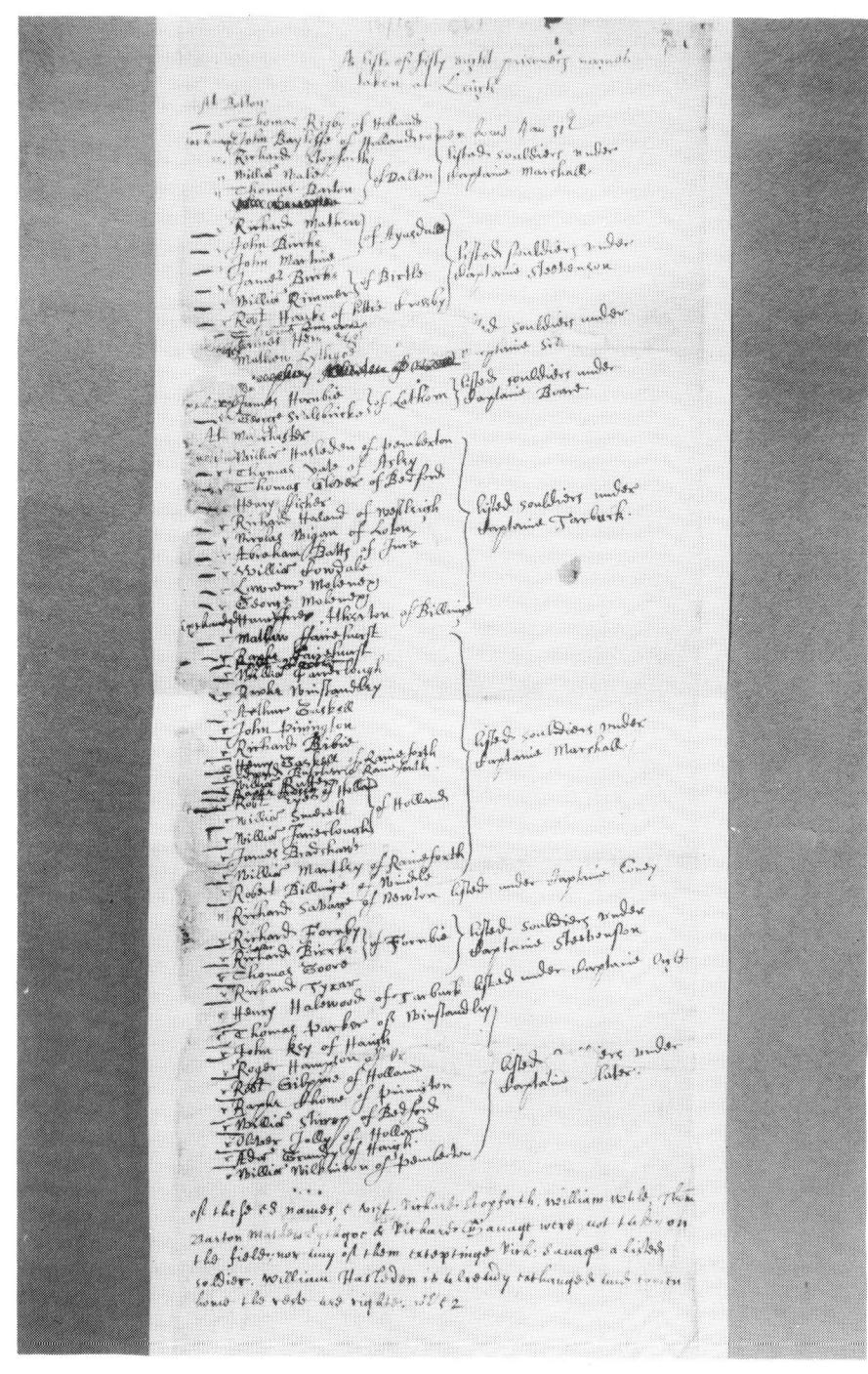

'A List of fifty-eight prisoners' names taken at Leigh': *this contemporary document lists the Royalists captured in December 1642 and held at Bolton (Anderton Papers).*

Miller, together with his horse and cart, had been commandeered by the Parliamentary forces to carry their ammunition, been captured along with them, but managed to convince the Royalists that he was not a volunteer.

At the end of 1642 both sides held on to what they had started with. During the winter of 1642-43 both forces were reinforced: the Royalists by the return of the veteran cavalry troop of Lord Molyneaux which had distinguished itself in early skirmishes around Oxford, while the Parliamentarians received the valuable addition of Sir John Seaton's fresh regiment and the renowned general Sir Thomas Fairfax.

Carefully the Earl of Derby marshalled his meagre resources, concentrating on his three front line towns protected by outposts. Wigan was the Royalist headquarters and was held by three infantry companies which should have provided 300 men, a troop of cavalry giving 100 more and 300 dragoons. Even here there were manpower shortages and Derby urged his three infantry captains, Barrow, Charnock and Chisnall to bring them up to full strength. To give warning against surprise attack several outposts containing about 20 men were established at Brindle, Ince, Hindley, Chowbent and Leigh under Captain Slater and Lieutenant Ranicar. The shortages of men were beginning to worry Derby and he urged all the neighbouring gentry to make a list of their tenants and then exercise and train them with weapons so that they could act as a reserve. Command at Wigan was given to a Scot, "Sergeant Major General" Blair. A war council to assist Blair consisted of the Mayor, William Forth, Sir William Gerrard, Mr Ogle, Mr Lloyd, Mr Anderton of Lostock, Mr Ashton of Chadderton and Mr Sherrington, together with the infantry captains. Lieutenant Woods was appointed town provost marshal in charge of military discipline, while Captain Orchard was to be Blair's adjutant and assist him in his administration. Thomas Pilkington was made 'scowte master' with instructions to ride out every night with five men and every day with two men "to make discoveries", reporting in person to Blair twice daily immediately on his return from reconnaissance. For this important and dangerous work Pilkington was paid 20s (£1) a day. Pilkington seems to have been indulging in a little private looting because Derby ordered him to produce any goods in his men's possession so that they could be valued, then either bought by the committee or kept by the scouts. William Pilkington was made "overseer of the work nowe in hand for fortifyinge of the towne" and for this he was paid 12d (5p) a day. Entrenchments were dug, earthen ramparts thrown up round the town and the gates and entrances strengthened. A small fort was built on Parson's Meadow near Adam Bridge and the lines of defense could be seen until 19th century colliery spoil heaps obliterated them.

A most difficult task was allotted to Henry Ogle, who was made Quartermaster General with the job of "bringinge provision to the Army at reasonable rates". In an early attempt at price-fixing it was suggested that food for the soldiers and fodder for their horses should be bought at 12d for 16 pounds of bread, 3d for a pound of butter, 2d for a pound of cheese and 2d for a store of hay, although it was admitted that later purchases would be at market rates.

Three soldiers of Captain William Houghton's company were billeted on William Wakefield, a Wigan panner (metalworker) and their 26 meals cost 7s. 7d. Sums like this could soon mount up as Captain Chisnall's account for only a fortnight proves:

		Number of Men	£. s. d.
Sunday	8th January	85	3. 3. 9.
Monday	9th January	88	3. 6. 0.
Tuesday	10th January	88	3. 6. 0.
Wednesday	11th January	91	3. 8. 3.
Thursday	12th January	89	3. 6. 9.
Friday	13th January	90	3. 7. 6.
Saturday	14th January	90	3. 7. 6.
Sunday	15th January	88	3. 6. 0.
Monday	16th January	92	3. 9. 0.
Tuesday	17th January	91	3. 8. 3.
Wednesday	18th January	91	3. 8. 3.
Thursday	19th January	90	3. 7. 6.
Friday	20th January	90	3. 7. 6.
Saturday	21st January	90	3. 7. 6.
			46. 19. 9. (14)

The destruction of many town records has robbed us of an insight into that indispensable twilight world of warfare - espionage. It undoubtedly went on locally during this period, and a fascinating glimpse is revealed when a suspected Parliamentarian spy was captured near Wigan on 13 January 1643. Margaret Hulme, wife of Edward Hulme, a Bolton fustian weaver, was arrested and questioned, having been intercepted carrying a letter from a Parliamentary agent in Warrington to a spymaster in Bolton and found to have £100 concealed on her person. During her interrogation she tried to explain by saying that she had travelled to Warrington on the previous Monday to see her husband, held prisoner there after his capture in the fight on Lowton Common, and had been asked by Mary Morris, daughter of John Morris of Bolton, to carry a letter to Mr Wooley of Warrington without knowing what the contents of the letter were. She further admitted that she travelled back from Warrington on the Thursday in the company of a Hindley man, William Aspull, a badger (travelling salesman); he had carried her basket on one of his pack horses. She had stayed overnight, free of charge, at his house before being picked up by a Royalist patrol in Hindley on the Friday morning. She denied all knowledge of the letter found in her possession and said that the money was from Mrs Wooley for John Morris.

The contents of the letter were quite damning. The top of the letter is missing with most of the addressee's name torn off but reads "Good Mr. N...." It was probably addressed to Norris (Morris) and is extremely revealing, giving figures of the Royalist strength and troop movements, the level of their morale and details of how far he (Wooley) could help behind enemy lines.

The writer (presumably Wooley) goes on to admit to being a little careless and almost giving himself away:

> "I have done my best endeavour to get the Papists put out of this towne tenn days since and was then in good hope to have prevailed in itt and to have likewise wrought some of the best of the town to have layd downe their Armes and submitted to the Parliaments forces but my good desires were att that tyme crossed and such a suspition is now growne upon me that I dare not be seene in any such business."(15)

He continues by stating that, if Parliament was to attack Warrington, he would do his best to undermine the defenders' cause from within; the attack, however, had better come soon because there were 800 soldiers, 300 armed townspeople and 80 dragoons in the town already, with a further 1,500 dragoons and 2,000 infantry expected to arrive soon. He then goes on to describe how he intended to betray the town:

> "If you give mee sure intelligence of your tyme I shall provide a gyde to lead you in. I can with ease guyde you such a way you may enter quickly and besides I have a meanes to make way to the magazine."

The writer was very confident that his letter would get through:

> "If you give mee any directions by this bearer I shall follow them in the best manner I can which yow may safly doe for shee is free from all suspition but unless you do so I shall not knowe how to carry my selfe."

However, the bearer was stopped and the letter with its incriminating contents intercepted. The Earl of Derby conducted the interrogation himself at his headquarters in Wigan. But it is not known what became of Margaret Hulme.

Chapter 4

Breakthrough

THE Parliamentarians launched the opening attack of 1643 when they broke through the Earl of Derby's left flank and captured Preston on 10 February 1643. This brilliant offensive was carried out by mostly fresh and untried troops strengthened by a nucleus of veterans. Far from giving in to this disaster the Earl of Derby decided that attack was the best form of defence and attacked Bolton. Blair issued a proclamation calling on all able-bodied men between the ages of 16 and 60:

> "to bee and appeare at the Towne of Wigan upon Monday next with their beste and complete armes, weapons and habilments of warre and likewise with provision of victuals".(16)

MAP 2 : BREAKTHROUGH : February - May 1643

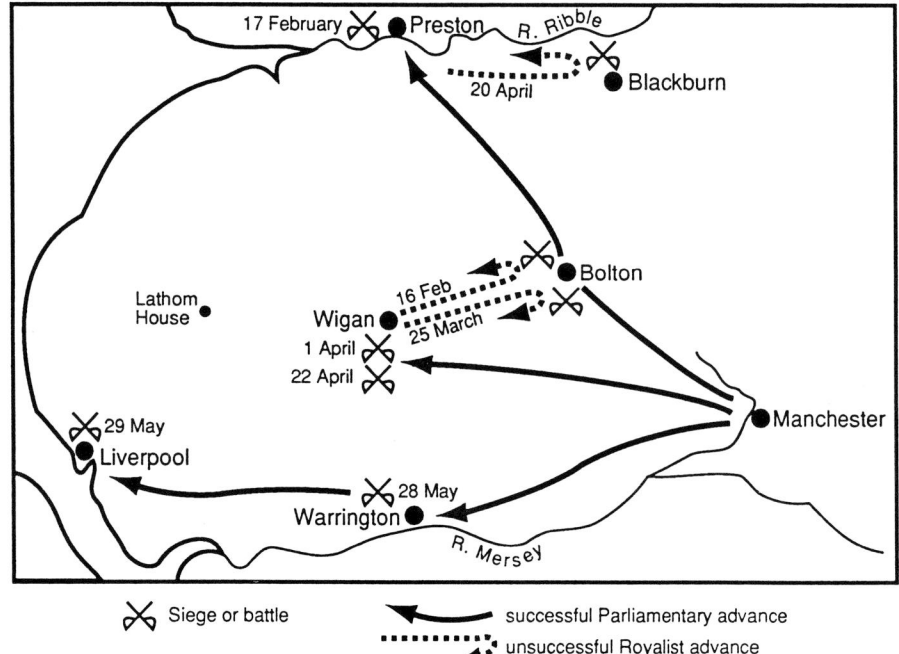

On 16 February the Royalists attacked Bolton. Now it was the Parliamentarians' turn to suffer a surprise attack, but they did not succumb to it. If Derby thought that Bolton would be an easy target because many of its defenders were still at Preston, he was sadly mistaken. Slowly the Royalists were pushed back, and news came that help was on the way for the defenders. Parliamentarian sympathisers from the countryside around Bolton together with 200 fresh soldiers from Manchester under Captain Radcliffe, all hurried towards the scene; before they arrived, however, the Royalists had slipped away, taking with them two or three cartloads of dead bodies and leaving behind about a dozen dead and mortally wounded.

On 28 March 1643, the Wigan garrison made another attempt to capture Bolton but were beaten off far more easily than before. The Parliamentarians then decided that they would settle accounts with Wigan once and for all, and mounted their biggest military operation of the war in Lancashire so far, against Derby's key position. On 1 April 1643 over 2,000 men, mostly musketeers, with some pikemen, and a small detachment of 200-300 cavalry, under two of their best leaders — Assheton and Holland — attacked Wigan. It had been assumed by the Royalists that Wigan was impregnable but it was not to prove so. After an hour's fighting Assheton's musketeers forced their way into the town at the Poolstock end. Most of the defenders scattered, but a small band barricaded themselves in the parish church overlooking the Market Place and, firing from the tower, killed more Parliamentarians than had been killed during the earlier part of the attack.

A real comedy then followed. While the Parliamentarians were trying to dislodge the last fanatical defenders from their refuge the news came that a Royalist relief column was approaching the town. A few Parliamentarian cavalry under Lieutenant-Colonel Rosworm left the town to reconnoitre. They found the Royalist reinforcements to consist of only three incomplete troops of cavalry, who retreated on the approach of the Parliamentarians. Rosworm returned to Wigan, only to find Colonel Holland gathering together the Parliamentarian troops and preparing to retreat. Rosworm was furious and tried to persuade Holland to stay, or at least take the prisoners and leave him with 500 musketeers and a troop of horse with which to finish the job. Holland agreed to stay until the church had been captured; after Rosworm had threatened to blow it up and given the beleaguered Royalists an hour to think about it, 86 in all came out and surrendered. While he was dealing with this fresh batch of prisoners Holland marched off with virtually the entire force, leaving Rosworm with only one company of musketeers. Those troops, seeing how outnumbered

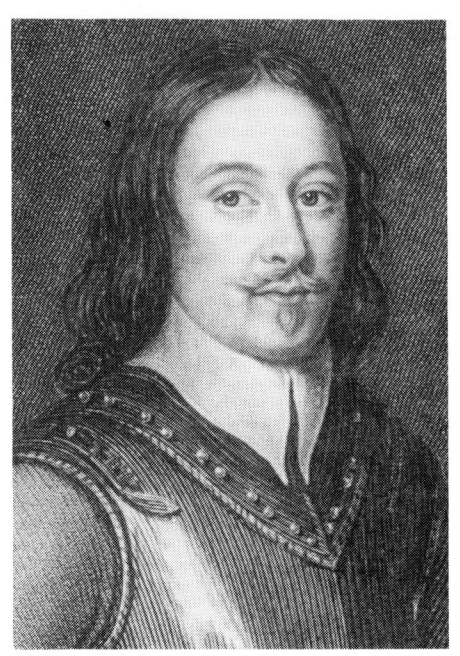

Sir Thomas Tyldesley, killed at the battle of Wigan Lane, 25 August 1651, and buried in Leigh parish church.

they were, also left, leaving Rosworm to deal with 400 prisoners, all the captured pikes and muskets and two large cannon, surrounded by hostile townspeople whose houses had just been ransacked! Rosworm ran for his horse, then rode for his life.

Wigan had been thoroughly plundered. The town had been considered to be the safest place to store money, jewellery, plate and other valuables; about £20,000 worth of goods, an enormous sum in those days, is said to have been stolen from the Moot Hall. The Cloth Hall was looted and great heaps of linen, wool and fustians littered the market place. The town records were thrown into the street and destroyed. The church was ransacked, its records also destroyed, its furniture wrecked and any contents of value stolen. It was a stunning blow from which the town took some years to recover. Lord Derby raced to Wigan as fast as he could, but on reaching Standish learned of the enemy's success and hurried departure, so made for Lathom House in preparation for the expected attack on it.

The end was in sight for the Lancashire Royalists and it came in an unlikely way and at an unlikely place. By 19 April 1643 Derby was making a move towards Blackburn with probably the largest force he ever raised in Lancashire during the civil wars — between 3,000 and 5,000 men.

Although Derby's army was huge by local standards, the quality was low. There were, it is true, 700 of his best cavalry and 700 good infantry, led by his top officers, including Molyneaux, Tyldesley and Hoghton; the bulk of the force, however, consisted of poorly armed and ill trained agricultural workers from the Fylde. Nevertheless, they outnumbered the Parliamentarians by about four to one. The Parliamentary commanders wanted to retreat, but the common soldiers were determined to fight. As the Royalist advance guard marched out of a dip in a narrow lane near Whalley they were met by a well-timed volley of musket fire which threw them into chaos. The advance guard — including the fearless Sir Thomas

20

Tyldesley — broke and ran, throwing the main body into disorder. The Parliamentarians gave a shout and charged them, starting a rout which lasted all of five miles back to the river. Some of the Royalist infantry never stopped running until they reached Preston. This little-known skirmish at Sabden Brook was the decisive battle of the Civil War in Lancashire. The King's cause was lost in the county.

Supporters of Parliament now gathered themselves for the final push. Once more Assheton appeared before Wigan with another huge force of 2,200 infantry and cavalry. On 22 April 1643 he occupied the town without meeting any resistance, the small Royalist garrison under Colonel Tyldesley having retreated to Lathom House. Assheton demolished the town's fortifications, burned the newly constructed gates and made the townsmen take an oath that they would never again take up arms against King and Parliament. This oath shows that the Parliamentary forces were fighting, not for a republic, but for joint government by monarch and parliament. On 27 May 1643 Warrington surrendered. By then Liverpool was already in Parliament's hands. Hornby and Thurland Castles were captured soon afterwards, leaving only Lathom House and the isolated Greenhalgh Castle in Royalist hands.

Chapter 5

Prince Rupert

MEANWHILE King Charles I had learned of the efforts of his loyal subjects in Wigan, and on 25 February 1644 he sent a letter addressed to the Mayor and Burgesses of the town which read:

> "Trusty and Wellbeloved Wee Greete you well. Whereas We have received particular information of the singular affection you have lately expressed in your great expense, approved fidelity, and indefatigable industry against the Rebels in those parts, we doe hereby return Our Royal Thanks for the same, and Assure you We will always remember your loyal and faithful Endeavours in Our service abovsayd upon all occasions for your advantage. And soe We bid you heartily Farewell. Given att our Court att Oxford the 25th of February in the eighteenth year of our reign."(17)

As for the Royalist leaders in Lancashire, Derby had retreated to his other stronghold, the Isle of Man, Tyldesley had joined Lord Newcastle in Yorkshire, while Molyneaux linked up with the Royalists at Chester. Derby's wife Charlotte de la Tremouille was left to defend his ancestral home, Lathom House. Charlotte was the grand-daughter of William, Prince of Orange. Like him she was a devout Protestant and was later to prove herself to be, when she defended her home against an army, a brave and courageous woman.

Lathom was not really a house. It was a castle, but unlike other medieval fortresses which had fallen to that new weapon of war — gunpowder — Lathom could be adapted for defence against artillery. The strong red sandstone building was surrounded by a wall two yards thick with nine towers at intervals along it, each capable of holding six cannons, and the only entrance through the wall was dominated by a huge gatehouse with double towers. Outside the wall a moat eight yards wide and two yards deep kept attackers from closing in. The house itself possessed a central tower, the Eagle Tower, which gave an excellent view of the surrounding area. Another point in Lathom's favour was its site — in a hollow surrounded by a low rise in the ground — described by John Seacome, an 18th century historian, as being 'like the palm of a man's hand'. Besiegers could not therefore bring direct artillery fire against the walls.

But Lathom's strongest asset was the character of the defenders. The Countess of Derby was fortunate that her devoted lieutenants – William Farmer (later killed at Marston Moor), William Farrington, Edward Chisenhall, Edward Rosthorn, Henry Ogle, Richard Fox and Molyneaux Radcliffe – were not only loyal and fanatical in her cause but, as will be seen, alert and enterprising. The garrison numbered 300, divided into six companies, and there were even 12 cavalrymen under William Kay.

In February 1644 a Parliamentary army some 2,500 strong, drawn mainly from Bolton and Manchester, arrived at Lathom House under the direction of Sir Thomas Fairfax, with four implacable Parliamentarian Commanders: Ralph Assheton, Robert Holland, John Moore and Alexander Rigby. On 28 February Fairfax requested the Countess to surrender. Negotiations were spun out until 11 March as Fairfax, Rigby, Assheton, a Colonel Morgan, and a Captain John Ashhurst all tried to persuade the wily but courageous Countess to surrender. They all left nonplussed by her demeanour and determination.

The siege began in earnest on 12 March 1644 with a bombardment of the house. First to be targeted was the outer wall, and efforts were made to make a breach for the besieging army to pour through. When this was found to be having no effect, attention was turned to the tower in an attempt to demoralise the defenders. The effect of this bombardment was to stir the garrison to action.

On 12 March Captain Farmer with 100 foot soldiers and 12 horsemen sallied out from the defences, killed several of the besiegers and took six of them prisoner. The following Sunday night Captain Chisenhale sallied out from the rear gate and put the Parliamentarians to flight. Meanwhile the besiegers fired cannon at the house, but most of the damage was done by a large mortar, loaded with grenades or huge stones. The Royalists then decided to make another night attack on the besiegers' camps. Captains Edward Chisenhall and Richard Fox were to lead the sortie, Captain Henry Ogle was to secure their safe retreat through the south gate, while Captain Rosthorne was to do the same at the east gate. Captain Radcliffe commanded marksmen on the top of the wall while Farmer held a reserve of men ready to reinforce anyone who needed it. At the appointed time (4 am on 26 April) Chisenhall sallied out of the east gate and into the fort where the Parliamentarians had sited their big guns. After a brief skirmish the besiegers fled, leaving their dead and wounded behind. Fox now came up in support and the combined force made for the south-east corner where the mortar was, chasing Parliamentarians out of the trenches as they advanced. The huge weapon was then lifted on to a home made sledge, and hauled triumphantly into Lathom House.

The siege dragged on for several weeks, during which time the defenders began to run short of food and ammunition. But their ordeal was almost over.

Back in April 1643 when Wigan had been so easily captured, the Countess had realised that unless help came from outside, the Royalist cause in Lancashire would be lost. So she wrote to the King's most flamboyant general, her cousin Prince Rupert, then fighting in the south of England:

> "My Lord—I have just received the disastrous news of the loss of Wigan six miles from this place. It has held out for only two hours having been panic-struck. My husband was twelve miles off and before he was ready to succour it, it was surrendered. In the name of God my lord take pity on us; and if you appear you can conquer it easily, and with much honour to your highness. Have pity on my husband, my children, and me who are lost forever if God and your highness do not take pity on us.
> I am my lord your very humble and obedient servant,
> C. DE LA TREMAILLE
>
> At Lathom 1 April 1643"(18)

Rupert intended to march to York which was besieged by Parliament's forces, and was persuaded to relieve Lathom House on the way. He reached Lancashire on 25 May 1644 and routed the Parliamentary garrison of Stockport, which had rashly marched out to give him battle. On hearing this Alexander Rigby ended the 18 week siege of Lathom House and made for Bolton as fast as he could. His force arrived on the evening of 27 May 1644, swelling the number of defenders to about 2,500. The next morning Prince Rupert's army, having bypassed Manchester on their march from Stockport, arrived outside the walls of the town with the obvious intention of attacking it.

Rupert sent the customary demand for surrender but the defenders replied by firing their cannons in defiance. The Royalists approached the town about 2 o'clock in the afternoon, and at once delivered an attack; after about half an hour's fighting, however, they were beaten off.

Rupert called together his senior officers and proposed another assault, this time with twice as many men. The Earl of Derby realised that unless Bolton was taken and its garrison killed or captured (and Manchester shortly afterwards he hoped) before Price Rupert moved on to relieve York, the siege of Lathom House would soon be resumed. So Derby requested to be allowed to lead the attack at the head of his own men.

After a quarter of an hour Derby broke into the town at the head of 200 handpicked soldiers.

Some cavalry were admitted to another part of the town through the treachery of one of the inhabitants, with the result that every Parliamentarian soldier caught between the two forces had to save himself as he might. The entire garrison was killed or captured, apart from a few senior officers and cavalry who got away, including the Wigan M.P. Alexander Rigby. What followed next is one of the most controversial episodes in the history of the Civil War. The Puritans and Parliamentarians spread the word that the victorious Royalists rampaged through the town looting, pillaging, and raping and murdering in cold blood not only the defeated and demoralised soldiers but also innocent civilians including women and children. The best-known of these claims appeared in the pamphlet:

> "An Exact Relation of the bloody and barbarous Massacre at Bolton-in-the-Moors in Lancashire, May 28, by Prince Rupert being penned by an Eye Witness admirably preserved by the gracious and mighty hand of God in that day of Trouble. Published according to Order. Printed by R.W. for Christopher Meredith. London. 22 August 1644."

The writer is thought to have been the Rev. John Tilsley, Vicar of Deane 1642-1662, an implacable and bigoted opponent of the King.

Naturally the Royalist accounts of the fighting differ from the above in

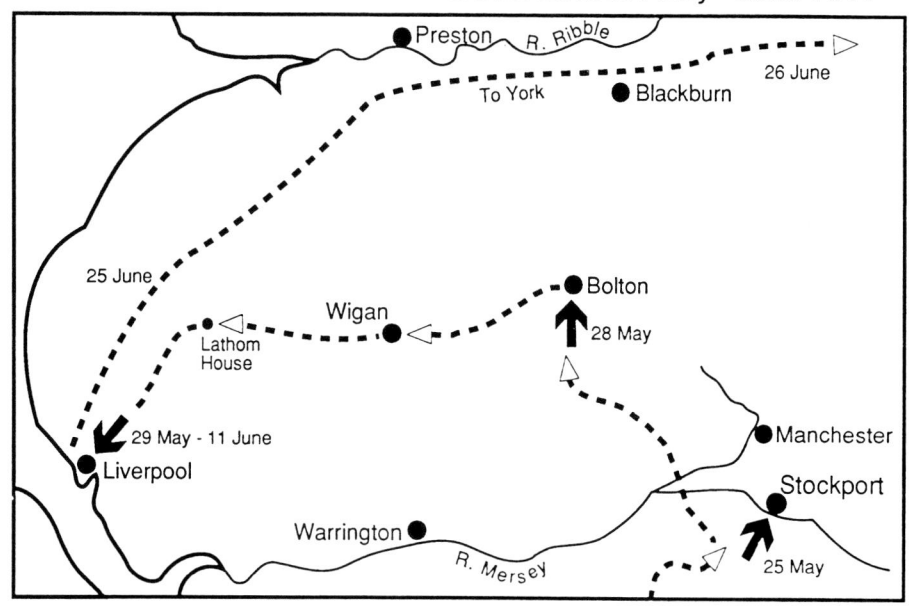

MAP 3 : PRINCE RUPERT IN LANCASHIRE : May - June 1644

that they do not mention the cold-blooded killing of women and children; one, however, does reveal that:

> "Rigby himself got away but left Two Thousand of his men behind him, most of which were slain upon the Place, the Prince forbidding to give Quarter to any person then in Arms."(19)

So the Royalists admit that many enemy soldiers found inside were killed and not given "quarter", that is the chance to surrender. This was often the option offered to defenders before a town was stormed — 'surrender or everyone inside will be killed' — partly as a threat or to bluff them into giving up, but also because it was known to be very difficult to keep control over soldiers who had forced their way into a town and suffered heavy losses doing so. Another Royalist account admits:

> "our foot entered the town over their works killing in the first heat of the action all who came in their way."(20)

Royalist justification of Rupert's conduct points to the killing of several Royalist prisoners on the town walls before Rupert's very eyes, in response to his initial request to surrender. This story too can be discounted as propaganda. As Prince Rupert left England before the end of the war and could not subsequently be brought to trial, the Parliamentarians turned their fury and lust for revenge on the Earl of Derby.

There is no proof that the Earl of Derby took part in the massacre which occurred during the capture of Bolton, except for one incident involving the death of Captain William Bootle. This soldier had once been Derby's servant, had joined up on the opposite side of the war and had played a prominent part in the siege of Lathom House. He had surrendered in return for his life being spared, only for the bargain to be broken. The Puritan pamphleteers, however, disagree as to his exact fate. One says that the Earl killed Bootle himself, another that Derby himself would not kill Bootle but allowed others to do so. In any event, this became the focus of the charges against Derby when he was captured six years later.

Rupert captured 22 regimental flags at Bolton, which he presented to the Countess of Derby in admiration of her courageous conduct during the siege of Lathom House, where they were draped around the walls of the banqueting hall. Rupert followed his trophies to Lathom House, pausing only in Wigan where he was met with wild enthusiasm and an official banquet held in his honour by the Mayor, Christopher Banckes, at a cost of £20. Rupert's next target was Liverpool where, not for the last time in his military career, he underestimated his opponents. The defenders fought fiercely, losing over half their numbers before surrendering.

Rupert marched to Lathom House, where he had the fortifications strengthened. Then he marched into Yorkshire by way of Preston, Clitheroe, Skipton and Otley en route to York which was under siege by the Parliamentarians. He out-manoeuvred the Parliamentary forces and pursued them to Long Marston, about seven miles from the city. There, at Marston Moor on 2 July 1644, the Parliamentary army turned on the Royalists and drove them from the field. In a single day all that Rupert had gained in a brilliant campaign was lost, and the Lancashire Royalists were once more left to fend for themselves. Lathom House was left alone to face a second siege, if anything more glorious than the first. The Earl and Countess of Derby were in the Isle of Man, and Farmer had been killed at Marston Moor, so Rawsthorne assumed command. Time, however, was against the gallant defenders of Lathom House. Supplies of food and ammunitions began to run low while casualties mounted as Rawsthorne lost men he could not replace. At the beginning of December 1645, after a siege lasting 15 months, Lathom House surrendered. The House, once "the pride and glory of Lancashire", was razed to the ground; not a single stone remains.

Chapter 6

Oliver Cromwell

FOLLOWING the Royalist defeat at Marston Moor on 2 July 1644 the Parliamentarians soon overran Lancashire once more and peace returned to the county. Charles surrendered to the Scots on 5 May 1646 in the hope that he could bargain for Scottish support against Parliament. The Scots handed him over to the English Parliament, but eventually an agreement was reached with him whereby they would help him regain his throne by force of arms, in return for his establishing the Presbyterian form of Church government in England.

After three years of peace Wigan found itself in the front line once again. On 8 July 1648 a 15,000 strong Scottish army under the Duke of Hamilton crossed the border near Carlisle, where they were joined by that ardent Royalist leader Sir Marmaduke Langdale with a fine little force of 3,000 infantry and 500 cavalry. Hamilton's cavalry were commanded by Sir John Middleton and the infantry by William Baillie. By 16 August 1648 Middleton, Callendar and the cavalry had reached Wigan, and Baillie's infantry were approaching Preston, their left flank protected by Langdale. On 17 August 1648 Cromwell's forces, although outnumbered two to one by Hamilton, swept down the Ribble valley to take the Scots in flank. The whole weight of Cromwell's attack fell on the unfortunate Langdale whose soldiers fought desperately for four hours, before breaking and fleeing towards Preston. Baillie's infantry were halfway across the River Ribble at Preston. Cromwell now attacked them with as many of his troops as he could collect. More vicious hand-to-hand fighting took place before the Roundheads captured the bridges and cut off the Scots from their base, most of Baillie's men having got across. By nightfall on 17 August 1648 about 1,000 of Hamilton's men had been killed, 4,000 captured, thousands of weapons lost, together with the supply wagons which had been abandoned by their civilian drivers.

Middleton ordered a night withdrawal, a difficult manoeuvre at the best of times, but given the appalling weather and low Scottish morale, this turned into a disaster. As Cromwell's exhausted troops slept where they had fought, the Scots infantry slipped away down the Standish road towards Wigan without being noticed. Middleton's cavalry, however, hurrying back from Wigan to the infantry's assistance, took the wrong path. At the Boar's Head Inn they followed the right hand fork in the road and galloped back to Preston via Chorley, while their infantry squelched down the Standish road. Middleton reached Darwen to find himself facing Cromwell's entire army. Turning round he made a fighting retreat all the way back to Wigan, skirmishing constantly with the Parliamentarian advance guard led by young Colonel Thornhaugh. In one clash Thornhaugh was mortally wounded by a Scottish lancer; as he lay by the roadside he asked his men to move aside so he "might see the rogues run".

Even now Hamilton still had 6,000 infantry and 3,000 cavalry outnumbering Cromwell's advance guard of 3,000 foot and 2,500 horse. Hamilton wanted to make a stand just north of Wigan but with morale low, powder wet, and match impossible to light, a battle was out of the question; covered by Middleton's cavalry, the infantry therefore continued towards Wigan.

A Royalist wrote later:

> "Next morning we appeared at Wigan Moor; half our number less than we were; most of the faint and weary soldiers having lagged behind; whom we never saw again."(21)

As darkness fell on 18 August 1648 the exhausted Scottish infantry stumbled into the town.

Cromwell and his men were too tired to go further. In his dispatch to the Speaker of the House of Commons he stated:

> "We lay that night in a field close to the enemy, and having marched twelve miles of such ground as I never rode in all my life the day being very wet."(22)

Although Cromwell did not know it, chaos reigned in Wigan. Scottish infantry, utterly demoralised and frantic with fear in case Cromwell's troops caught up with them, staggered through the town pilfering and stealing whatever they could.

About midnight Sir James Turner, who commanded the infantry rearguard, was marching through the Market Place in the centre of Wigan when some of his own cavalry caught him up and rode frantically past. Thinking that Cromwell's cavalry could not be far behind he halted his brigade, faced about, and formed them up in a body shoulder to shoulder, pikes levelled to repulse any pursuers. When a cavalry regiment appeared Turner recognised it as one of their own and ordered his men to open up and let it through. By this time his men were paranoid with fear and refused, even attacking and wounding him. He rode over to the cavalry and ordered them to charge the pikemen, but seeing the pikes pointing at them, they too refused. He then rode to the rear of the cavalry and cried out that Cromwell's men had arrived. The ruse was successful. The cavalry rode forward, most of the infantry threw down their pikes and ran into the houses, or the yards and alleys that lead off the market place, while those who stood their ground were trampled beneath the horses' hooves. Turner, a quick-witted and brave officer, then ordered drums to be beaten to call his men together. Before they could reassemble, however, the Scots looted the town; small wonder that the townspeople were glad to see them go.

Part of the Royalist forces were still well ahead of Cromwell's main body, with time to choose their own place to make a stand — on a slight slope where a stream crossed the road at Red Bank, Winwick, some three miles north of Warrington. Here they put up a determined fight until eventually they broke and ran, some 2,000 being taken prisoner and about 1,000 killed. The remnant of the army reached Warrington where they appeared to be ready to defend the bridge. But as soon as the Parliamentarians arrived their commander, Baillie, sent a message to Cromwell suggesting terms of surrender. Cromwell agreed to spare the Royalists' lives and to treat them civilly, if they would lay down their arms; this they did.

Cromwell remained in Lancashire for a few days, leaving the pursuit of Hamilton's tattered remnants to the local Cheshire and Staffordshire gentry and to fresh Parliamentary troops hastening northwards. He seems to have rested his tired troops in and around Wigan, from where he kept in touch with the military situation:

> Wigan, 23 August 1648
> "Gentlemen — I have intelligence even now come to my hands that Duke Hamilton with a wearied body of Horse is drawing towards Pontefract . . . as not daring to continue in those counties whence we have driven him the country people rising in such numbers and stopping his passage at every bridge.
> Major General Lambert with a very considerable force pursues him at the heels. I am marching northwest with the greatest part of the army where I shall be glad to hear from you. I rest,
> Your very affectionate friend and servant,
> OLIVER CROMWELL."[23]

The three days running fight from Preston through Wigan to Warrington is usually referred to as the Battle of Preston and has not been given much prominence in the history books. It was, however, one of the most significant battles in the history of England. It removed the last hopes of outside assistance for the King; on 30 January 1649 he was executed.

MAP 4 : CROMWELL IN LANCASHIRE : August 1648

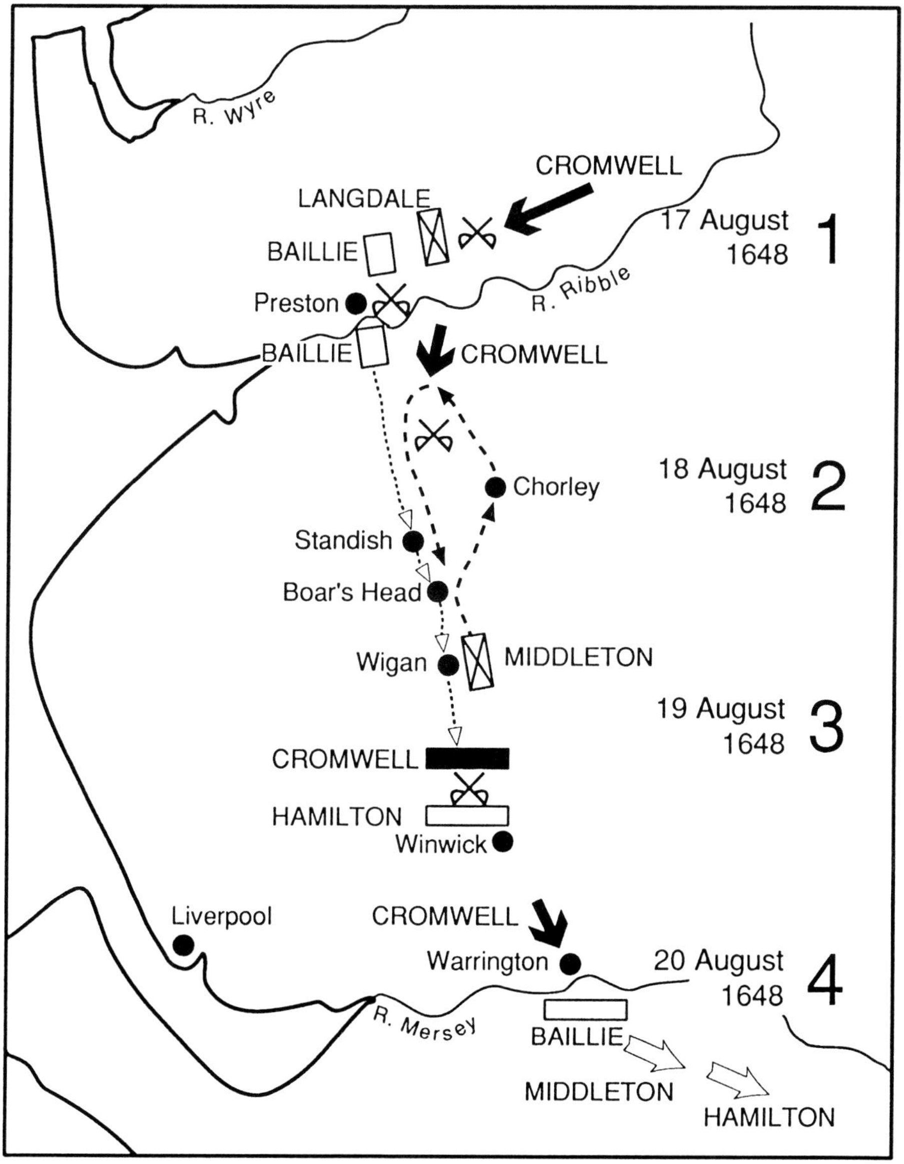

Parliamentary forces
Parliamentary forces
Royalist cavalry
Royalist infantry

Chapter 7

The Battle of Wigan Lane

ENGLAND had not seen the last of civil war – neither had Wigan. In June 1651 a Scottish army invaded England for the second time in three years, by the same route as before, this time with the young King Charles II at its head. By August 14 it had reached Wigan, and the King spent the night at Bryn Hall, the home of Sir William Gerard. The Earl of Derby had landed on 15 August 1651 at the mouth of the River Wyre, near the site of the modern port of Fleetwood, in seven ships carrying 60 cavalry and 300 foot soldiers. He had an interview with the King near Nantwich on 17 August and then returned to Lancashire. By 23 August Derby was in Preston with a force of about 1,500 men.

Meanwhile Colonel Robert Lilburne, having made a forced march from Cheshire, arrived at Wigan on 21 August. Finding the town empty of the enemy he advanced to Preston. Here, while his horses were grazing, a surprise attack caught Lilburne off guard; his soldiers, however, rallied and in the end chased the Royalists back to Preston, killing and taking prisoner about 30 while losing only two men. That night a fresh company of infantry arrived from Liverpool, together with two more which had marched from Chester on hearing of a Royalist uprising in Lancashire. Lilburne would have preferred to wait for Cromwell's veteran regiment which was reported to be at Manchester, but when Derby marched towards Wigan, he was forced to follow him in case the Earl got away. There was now the danger that Cromwell's infantry regiment, marching alone from Manchester, would be caught isolated by Derby's cavalry force and wiped out. Lilburne followed Derby southwards from Preston and was amazed when, on reaching Wigan, he saw the Royalists lined up across the road ready to give battle. Lilburne would have preferred to ride round the town to link up with the infantry marching from Manchester, but he was forced to fight.

MAP 5 : MOVEMENTS LEADING TO THE BATTLE OF WIGAN LANE : August 1651

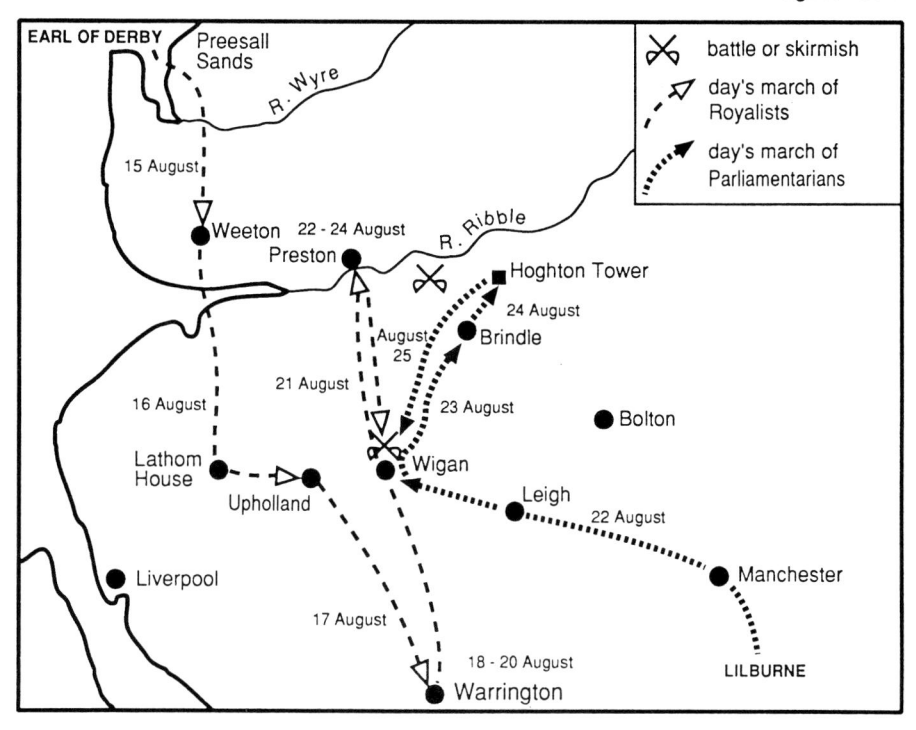

    The battle took place in Wigan Lane, between Mab's Cross at the outer end of Standishgate and Leyland Mill Lane near the present Cherry Gardens. The area then consisted of fields bounded by hedges with only one or two cottages, while the road was just a dirt track. Although it only lasted about an hour, the battle was an extremely severe encounter. Both sides were evenly matched in numbers. Lilburne had his own veteran cavalry regiment 600 strong with another 50 dragoons and about 30 more cavalry from Liverpool plus the two infantry regiments numbering 600. Derby had slightly more infantry, 800, but although they were all experienced individuals there had been no time to train them to fight together and Derby placed them in the rear. The Earl divided his cavalry into two units of about 300 each, commanding the van himself, and assigning the rear to Sir Thomas Tyldesley.
    At first the Royalists appeared to have the advantage, driving the Parliamentary forces back almost to Leyland Mill Lane. Again and again the Royalist cavalry charged but the opposing combination of veteran cavalry and carefully concealed well-led musketeers proved too much. Slowly the Royalists were driven back towards Wigan. Sir

Thomas Tyldesley's horse was shot from under him and as he tried to escape through a hedge he was shot in the back. So perished one of the most gallant soldiers of the war. Although his house was at Myerscough, near Garstang, where he had been Keeper of the King's Forest, Tyldesley also owned Morleys Hall, Astley and so he was buried in Leigh parish church where his grave can be seen today. In 1677, Alexander Rigby of Layton, Tyldesley's standard-bearer at the battle, erected the stone pillar in Wigan Lane, which marks the spot near which the gallant Royalist was killed. Several other high ranking officers were also killed, among them Colonel Boynton, Major Chester and Major Trollope; Lord Widdrington died of his wounds during the night. Widdrington, Boynton and Trollope were buried in Wigan church yard and although the site of their graves is lost their entries in the burial register can still be seen. About 300 soldiers were killed and over 400 captured together with all their weapons, baggage and supplies.

The Earl of Derby, wounded a number of times in the arms and shoulders, managed to escape into Wigan where he hid until darkness fell in the Dog Inn, Market Place. Among the booty captured by the victors were his three cloaks with stars, his George, his Garter (all

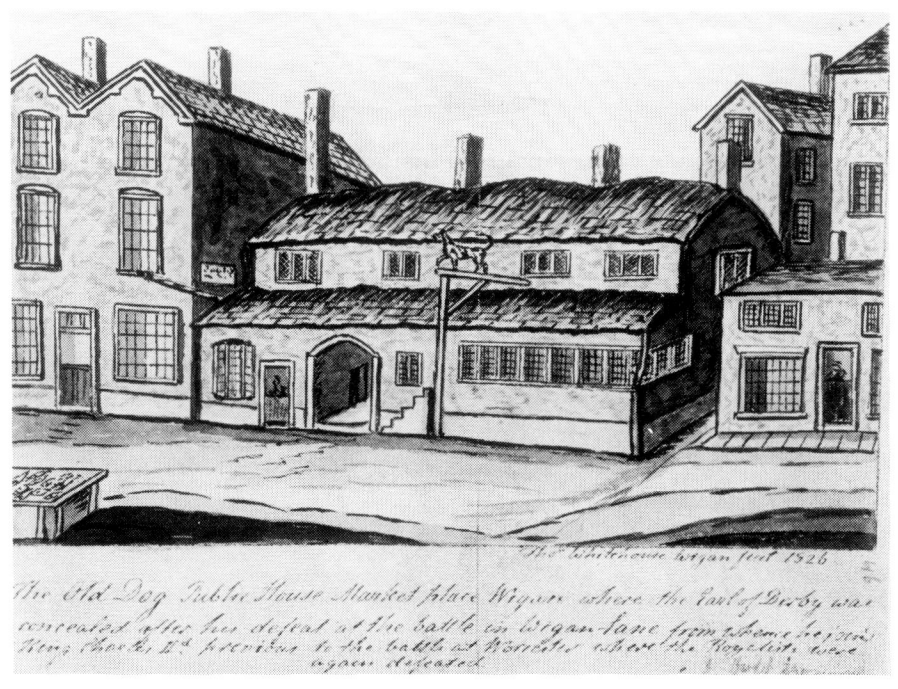

Watercoloured drawing by Thomas Whitehouse (1826) of the Old Dog, Market Place, where the Earl of Derby is said to have hidden after the battle of Wigan Lane.

insignia of a Knight of the Garter) and other personal belongings. The fur hat which he had worn over a steel helmet was afterwards picked up on the battlefield and found to have 13 sword cuts in it. During the night Derby, his aide Colonel Roscarrock and two servants, slipped away and rejoined the King just in time to take part in the Battle of Worcester on 3 September 1651, in which the Royalists were defeated once more. Surviving the battle, Derby, Lord Lauderdale and about 20 others, having broken away from a party of about 700 Royalists who were being harried by Parliamentarians near Nantwich, accidentally came across a lone Parliamentary officer named Oliver Edge. To Edge's amazement, they dismounted and surrendered to him. On 1 October 1651 the Earl was tried at Chester, and sentenced to death. He spent his last night at the King's Arms, Leigh (formerly situated behind the present Town Hall). Just after 12 o'clock on Wednesday 15 October 1651 he was executed in Bolton Market Place. According to contemporary chroniclers the scaffold was made from timber from Lathom House and erected at the spot where Captain William Bootle had been killed having been promised that his life would be spared. Derby maintained to the end that he was not responsible for his death.

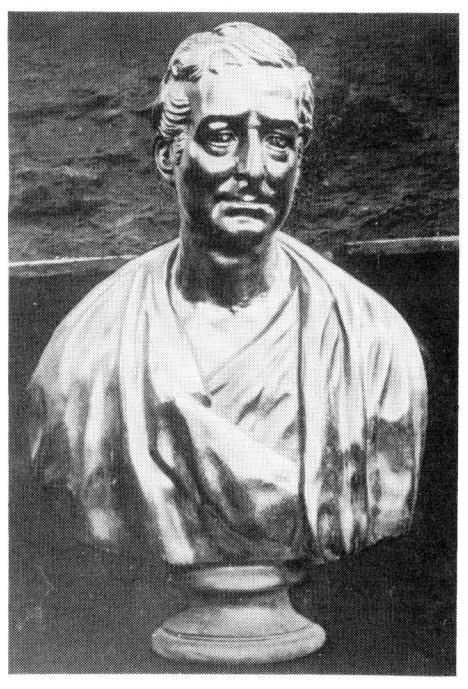

Bust of the Earl of Derby, executed at Bolton, 15 October 1651.

Chapter 8

Aftermath

WAR had left Wigan a battered and broken place. Among the fragments of documents which have survived are some pathetic entries. The plight of wounded soldiers, for example, could be desperate:

> "whereas it appeareth to this court that John Hatton and William Withington born within the parish of Leigh and beeing listed soldiers under Captain Chaddocke and in their service for king and parliament have endured much labour and pains and performed their duties carefully and readily and in the same service have received many and greevous wounds in their arms and legs and other places of their bodies whereby they are maymed and become soe impotent and poore that they are not able to subsist but exposed to extreme poverty."(24)

Looting was an accepted military activity in the 17th century; the Earl of Derby issued a general order in an attempt to regulate it, but it is difficult to know how successful it was:

> "That no man shall offer to plunder without direction having the officer with him; as also that whosoever shall plunder shall bring in the goods taken to the end they may be disposed for the public good and those that take pains therein may be rewarded according to the discretion of the commissioners."(25)

This is a very revealing paragraph about the military practices of those times.

One of the most frequent inconveniences the civilians faced was the billeting (usually forced) of soldiers from both armies, because so often householders never received the payment due to them. Even several years after the fighting was over Wigan citizens were still petitioning the Court Leet in often vain attempts to obtain recompense, having provided overnight food and lodgings for the soldiers:

> "5th October 1650. To the right worshipfull mr maior, his brethren and burgesses of the burrough of Wigan the humble petition of James Rigby weaver. Sheweth that for the souldiers troopers under the command of Colonel Bethell, John Standish late bailiff received and took from your petitioner as much hay as your petitioner might have had ii Li iis [£2.10p] for the same and what strawe for bedding of horses worth is [5p] and for that your petitioner had never satisfaction for the said haye and strawe."(26)

Bethell had been stationed in Wigan during 1648 and two years later the bill had still not been paid.

Even the high point of the war so far as Wigan was concerned — the banquet held in honour of Prince Rupert — had not been paid for 20 years later!

> "1 October 1664. To the worshipfull the Maior, Aldermen and Burgesses att this leet assembled.
> The petition of William Browne.
> Sheweth that your petitioners late father was balife of this Borrowe in the year 1644 when Prince Ruperts Army marched through this towne att which tyme your said petitioners father and James Crucke then also Baylife did by the direction of the then mayor provide for the said Prince a Banckett and other Necessary but in regard of the tymes which then insued the said money for the same Banckett was not paid in all amounting to twenty Markes or upwards and in Regard that it hath pleased god to restore us into such a condition Nowe that the same may be justly expected."(27)

Poor weather conditions added to farming difficulties. Disease too began to spread. Plague, which had been dormant for years, suddenly broke out again at this inopportune time. In 1648 conditions were so bad that public meetings were banned and the fortnightly Wigan Court Leet was not held between 4 February 1649 and 1 September of the same year. The epidemic was rife as the parish register of Wigan church shows:

	Plague Victims
February 1649	0
March 1649	16
April 1649	36
May 1649	11
June 1649	6
July 1649	8
August 1649	0

For Wigan there was one lasting effect of the Civil War. On the restoration of the monarchy the new King, Charles II, rewarded Wigan for its adherence to the Royalist cause. In the summer of 1660 the Mayor wrote to Charles reminding him of his father's promise to reward the town for its loyalty, and petitioned to have the Duchy of Lancaster court transferred to Wigan from the town of Lancaster. The King replied in a letter dated 14 July 1660 that he would do so "if it were not prejudicial to the king's service"; nothing, however, became of it. In 1662, however, the King granted Wigan a new charter, together with the privilege of having a ceremonial sword carried before the Mayor in all processions. This in effect knighted the town.

Chapter 9

Conclusion

WHAT was the war about? Was it to decide who should rule the country, King or Parliament? Was it to decide what should be the official form of religion for the people of England? Was it an attempt to secure political representation by a previously excluded class of people? Was it all of these? Or was it more?

An interesting document has survived, the first draft of a letter from the Earl of Derby to King Charles I, written on 14 February 1644, when the Royalist cause in Lancashire seemed lost. Here is part of it:

> "We hope the many troubles of this Country have been already represented to you whereby your Majestie may be assured of our faithful endeavours to the best of our power to serve you in.
> Besides the general disaffection of a great part hear hath so disabled us that it is not possible we can now continue long without some speedy help.
> We are willing still to the last drop of blood or while we can make any resistance to stand it out.
> We suspect the common people rebel (as in most places in this Kingdom) will if not timely curbed become Lords over us."(28)

It is not known whether the later version retained these sentiments or even if it was sent at all; this first draft, however, reveals a depth of thought beyond the immediate urgency of the situation, desperate as that was.

Too often subsequent historians have stressed the religious and economic causes of the war. As the elections in Wigan showed there was a substantial body of people who had no say in the running of the country but who nevertheless wished to take part, either through influencing those already enfranchised or by obtaining the franchise themselves. The Earl of Derby realised this when others in positions of greater authority perhaps did not.

References

(1) *Wigan Court Leet Rolls*

(2) ibid

(3) ibid

(4) Quoted in HARDWICK, Charles: *History of the Borough of Preston.* (1857) p.168

(5) ibid p.169

(6) *Anderton Papers* (Wigan Archives)

(7) ibid

(8) ibid

(9) ibid

(10) ibid

(11) ibid

(12) ibid

(13) ibid

(14) ibid

(15) ibid

(16) ibid

(17) Quoted in HAWKES, Arthur J: *Wigan's Part in the Civil War* (1932) p.118

(18) Quoted in BAINES, Thomas: *History of the Commerce and Town of Liverpool* (1852) p.306

(19) Quoted in SCHOLES, James C: *History of Bolton* (1892) p.413

(20) ibid p.416

(21) Quoted in Hardwick, op.cit. p.195

(22) Quoted in Hardwick, op.cit. p.189

(23) Quoted in Hardwick, op.cit. p.195

(24) *Anderton Papers*

(25) ibid

(26) *Wigan Court Leet Rolls*

(27) ibid

(28) *Anderton papers*

WIGAN HERITAGE SERVICE

The Metropolitan Wigan area has a long and rich history, and interest in our local heritage has never been higher. Wigan Heritage Service, comprising the Archives, Museums and Local History services, seeks to preserve this heritage and to interpret it to as wide an audience as possible. The Heritage Service has major public outlets in Wigan and Leigh.

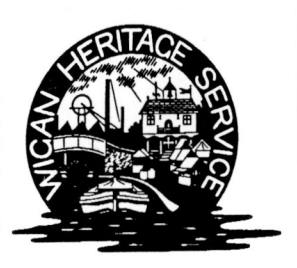

THE HISTORY SHOP

This new heritage development is located in the Old Library, Rodney Street, Wigan — a splendid Alfred Waterhouse building of 1878. The History Shop is, we believe, the first of its kind in Britain. It offers the following attractions:

- a state of the art display, telling the story of the Wigan area from the earliest times to the present day
- a temporary display area, in which the Service's art collection figures prominently
- a study/research centre, incorporating the Wigan Local History collection and a genealogical centre of excellence
- a small retail outlet, selling a range of heritage-related merchandise, including books, photographs and quality souvenirs
- a meeting/lecture room, with a programme of public lectures and displays; this room is also available for hire by local societies and groups.

The History Shop has something for everyone — young or old, local or non-local. For further information, please telephone **(0942) 828128**.

THE ARCHIVES AND LOCAL HISTORY SERVICE, LEIGH

Original archival documents for the Metropolitan Wigan area can be consulted in the Archives Service searchroom in Leigh Town Hall. These include records of churches, schools, societies and businesses, official council archives, papers of local families, estates and individuals and copies of census returns. For further information, please telephone **(0942) 672421 ext 266**.

Leigh Local History Service operates from the Turnpike Centre, Leigh Library. The collection includes local books and pamphlets, maps, photographs, newspapers and copies of parish registers and census returns. To find out more, telephone **(0942) 604131**.

Other Heritage Service attractions include Astley Green Colliery, Hindley Museum and The Stables Centre, Haigh Country Park. For further details of these, telephone **(0942) 828128**.

REMEMBER — *You can be of service to the Heritage Service. If you have any items in which you think we might be interested, please do not hesitate to contact us, on* **(0942) 828128**.